Lynn's Legacy

Mind, Body & Spirit

practices for a *better* life

Jenna.

Peace always.

Christa Johnson

Christa Johnson, MD

Center for Mind Body Health

Center for Mind Body Health
www.CenterForMindBodyHealth.com or
www.cfmbh.com

First Paperback Edition published in 2008

ISBN   978-0-9820819-0-7

Library of Congress Control Number: 2008907755

Copyright permissions

Excerpts from Robert A. Emmons, Joanna Hill, *Words of Gratitude for Body and Soul*, Pennsylvania, Templeton Foundation Press, 2001. Used in Gratitude Meditation (CD#1, track#3) with permission.

DEDICATION

To my dear friends Lynn Cutter and Dr. Beth Thomas, whose lives, illnesses and ultimate deaths broke my heart wide open, allowing me to experience the world on a deeper level, and to recognize what really matters.

To Dr. Patti Croft, Sharon Hague, Ruthanne Vargus, June Monteiro, Dr. Maria Delbecarro, Bob Whitney, Michelle Cruise, Pat Backus, Terri Gomes, Gretchen Spangler, Karen Brady and Patty Stuck for always being there to show me that in friendship, unconditional love is possible. .

To Dr. Barbara Greene, my teacher, spiritual guide, healing angel and mother of my heart.

To Linda Phelan whose awe-inspiring work with women with cancer at her Healing Coop proves, yet again, that things of great beauty and enormous value can come from one's own tragedy, and also for designing the beautiful cover for this book.

To my mentor and role model, Dr. Merle Ingraham, for showing me just how loving and wonderful a physician can be and for believing that I could follow in his footsteps.

To "Uncle Dave" Johnson, a true gift to my family, in whose presence not having fun or being unhappy is inconceivable.

To my dad, Earl, whose influence encouraged a work ethic that has made my medical career and this book possible.

To my mom, Claire, whose physical, emotional and addiction challenges in life made me recognize my own life's purpose. If I can teach what she never understood, that happiness is a conscious choice; both of our lives will have been worthwhile.

To my brother, Skip, whose unique sense of humor keeps us all from taking ourselves too seriously.

To my husband, Doug, for his enduring love and support, for being the best possible dad to our children and for bringing me and my right brain back to planet Earth only when absolutely necessary.

And to my children, Anna, Mike, Sarah (Matt, Kate, Alex and Hilary), for pushing me beyond what I thought was my limit of love, worry, joy, frustration… mostly love. For better or worse, they are far and away my best teachers.

ACKNOWLEDGEMENTS

To my editor, Susan Siegmann, Tim Snider and Nathaniel Lanzer from BookMasters, Inc. for all their help with the publication of this book.

To Peg Baim, Dr. Herbert Benson, and all the teachers at the Benson-Henry Institute for Mind Body Medicine whose inspired teachings and research have affirmed the knowledge that has been in my heart all along.

To Dr. Brian Weiss, Lama Surya Das, Jack Kornfield, Sharon Salzberg, Pema Chodron, Dr.Carolyn Myss, Dr.Norman Shealy, Dr. Bernie Siegel, Dr. Christiane Northrop, Rev. Wayne Muller, Martin Rossman, Ram Dass, Joan Borysenko, Dr. Larry Dossey, Thich Nhat Hanh, Sylvia Boorstein, and His Holiness Dalai Lama whose books lectures and stories have touched, inspired and provided the basis for my own work.

And especially to Jon Kabat Zinn whose tenacity in working within the traditional University of Massachusetts Medical School, my alma mater, was awe-inspiring to say the least, and was crucial in the process of bringing these teachings to our patients.

CONTENTS

HOW TO USE THIS PROGRAM

First, you need to read this book with a CD player close at hand as the recorded meditations arc crucial to the process of learning meditation. You must also resist the urge to do as I have done so many times with audio programs, which is to just listen to the tapes or CDs without benefit of reading the material in the book. This program is designed to teach you meditation; a skill that I guarantee will help you with every aspect of your life.

In order for the program to have maximum impact, it is important that you read each section and then listen to the associated guided meditation. The book will give you the background needed for an intellectual understanding, while the guided meditations will bring it right to your heart where the most profound learning takes place.

It would also be helpful to do this program in a place where you feel comfortable, at peace and won't be disturbed for a period of time. Like meditation, reading this book and listening to the guided meditations will be most effective if you can put aside enough time to read a whole section, do the associated meditation and then allow time to digest what you have learned. **Do not listen to the meditations while you are driving!** They are designed to put you in a deep state of relaxation - not a great idea when you are behind the wheel.

I have been a physician for over 25 years and I know of nothing more helpful for your body, mind and spirit than spending a few moments each day just being and learning to listen to your own inner wisdom. To answer any question or solve any problem that you have, you need to look no further than within yourself.

Meditation helps you to look at and learn from your own life, something we in western culture rarely take the time to do or fully understand. Taking the time to become acquainted with your inner being through meditation allows you to take over where your doctor leaves off. Leave the physical cures to your physician; your healing is up to you. It is my sincere hope that this program will help you to do just that.

LYNN'S LEGACY

CHAPTER ONE

Lynn...

My dear friend Lynn was diagnosed with ovarian cancer 10 years ago; she passed away two years later. Devastated as any 40-year-old woman would be at such news, in true Lynn form, she faced her illness with iron will and determination, pretty much as she lived her life. Lynn had a very strong personality. No shrinking violet, she never had a problem with making her opinion known. In her presence, there was never any doubt as to who was in control. She was a force of nature and my approach to her was just to sit back, watch and learn.

One could never accuse Lynn of being a touchy-feely emotional type, but anyone who knew her benefited from her core of pure gold. Like the sun coming up each morning, Lynn could be counted on to help anyone in need. She had an uncanny sense of another's distress, often showing up to lend support just when it was needed. I can still see her floating down my street one day many years ago, taking my children and me in hand, wordlessly feeding us, handing me a glass of wine, and being there on the very day another friend, Beth, was diagnosed with stomach cancer. Lynn never met Beth and didn't even know the news I had gotten that day, but somehow she felt my sadness and was there. This was a typical scenario in the lives of those who were fortunate enough to have this woman as a friend.

Lynn definitely saw herself as the helper, and even with a life threatening illness, would be a reluctant helpee. So it was both a shock and an honor when she asked me to go through the journey of her illness with her. Even she needed someone's support through this time. But on some level, Lynn would use the occasion of her cancer and ultimate death to do something good for the world... through me.

As one would expect, Lynn tackled her illness with the indomitable spirit that defined her. However, she was diminished by a medical system that, though unsurpassed in the technology required for curing bodies, was unaware of the importance of recognizing and validating her spirit. In fact, in most medical circles, any reference to the spirit in healing is thought to be nonsensical at best, a mere opiate for the unsophisticated masses. The mandate of western medicine is clear and that is to do whatever is required to keep the physical body alive. This is an honorable and worthy goal, to be sure. In my opinion, being a western trained physician myself, we do this as well as if not better than, anyone else in the world.

Cancer therapies have provided the means for miraculous cures; unimaginable a few decades ago, and yet something inherent in the process causes irreparable damage to the being that lives in the body.

Over the months of her state-of-the-art treatment, I watched Lynn's most defining feature—her self-assured, powerful spirit—wither. It became my personal mandate to figure out why. A few weeks before her death, Lynn told me that her illness and ultimate demise would be worthwhile if I would take what I learned from it and do something to change the practice of medicine. Undaunted by the enormity of this request, Lynn made it clear this was the direction my medical career would take. Who was I to say no?

So, what does a serious illness do to a person? The obvious answer can be stated in one word: FEAR—fear of the pain and suffering, fear of the expense, fear of the toll on loved ones, fear of treatment itself—and the penultimate human fear of all, fear of death. Surely, this alone would be enough to crush the spirit of most people, but not Lynn. She marched into this diagnosis and treatment with the same resolve as she marched through her life, always the woman with a purpose. She was as in control of the situation as any person could be; until, as so often happens, her wishes and control over her life and treatment were usurped by the brilliant and well-intentioned traditional western medical system.

In the course of cancer treatment, complicated protocols based on extensive and scientific study leaves no room for an individual patient's wants or concerns. Lynn's inquiries about complementary therapies (not to replace traditional practice but as adjuncts) were dismissed as unproven and therefore worthless. Sadly, patients are rarely given any active role, much less say, in their treatment, with the expectation being total abdication of control to the doctor. Control was central to the person Lynn was and having it taken away was a major impediment to her healing.

4

Despite how this may be perceived, this book is in no way an indictment of the western medical establishment, of which I have been a part for over two decades. Despite Lynn's wish that I do something to change medicine, I have come to realize that, except perhaps to open the minds of a few traditional medical fundamentalists, medicine does not need changing. It is quite remarkable just as it is and we should all be grateful for all that it offers.

What is needed, however, is to teach a patient that even in illness or any other hardship, taking control of one's own mind and spirit is possible and makes all the difference. Western thought and culture indicates that our minds and bodies are separate entities and that we are passive victims to all that befalls us. The truth is the impact that our thoughts and emotions have on our physiology is huge and we have a lot more control than we think we do. Extensive research over the last few decades has shown just how powerful our minds are; but this concept has yet to be given the place that it deserves in traditional western medicine.

With all due respect to western medical research, protocols and treatment, engaging not only our patients' bodies but also their minds and spirits gives them the best possible shot at whole-person healing of which physical cure is only, though not necessarily the most important, part. In fact, a person's attitudes, emotions and psyche are the most powerful allies that a physician has to insure the best possible outcome.

In retrospect, the needs and questions that Lynn had for me during her "journey" through cancer and death completely changed my life, career and direction. To answer her questions to the best of my ability, I read dozens of books and reached into the depths of my being through my own meditation practice to help her through her final life's process. Although she never achieved a physical cure, I am certain that the introspective work that Lynn did as her life was ending healed her on a deep level. In some uncanny and inexplicable way, I know she shared what she loved to call her "journey" with me so that I could teach this to you.

This is Lynn's Legacy.

CHAPTER TWO

Why a Holistic Approach?

We have all heard of holistic medicine. As I see it, holistic medicine is an all-encompassing medicine that takes into consideration everything that makes up a human being—body, mind and spirit. It should not be considered alternative, but rather complementary to traditional medicine as it needs to embrace all that western medicine has to offer as well as practices including mind body medicine, acupuncture, massage, energy medicine and others. What further differentiates holistic from traditional medicine is the understanding that each individual needs to be empowered to make whatever decisions are best for him or her.

Traditional medicine focuses on the physical causes of illness. Bacteria and viruses cause infections, abnormally growing cells cause cancer, excess stomach acid causes ulcers, physical injury causes back pain, etc. While accepting this to be true, holistic medicine takes a broader view of what causes illness and what maintains health.

It would be foolhardy indeed not to embrace the obvious physical causes of one's illness. But a more holistic approach understands that in order for physical abnormalities to take place, conditions in an individual's body must be just right for the germs, abnormal cells or physical pain to thrive. These conditions may be physical, but may indeed have their origins in emotional, psychological or even spiritual realms. Louis Pasteur said, "It is not the germ but the sort of culture on which it falls that determines whether or not an individual develops a disease when exposed to germs." How else can we explain that during a flu epidemic, only a small proportion of people actually get the flu?

Traditional and holistic treatments of illness are quite different. Traditional medicine uses physical means to treat the physical abnormalities of the physical body. Antibiotics, pain medicines, chemotherapy, surgery, and radiation are the mainstays of traditional treatment. Although there has been some acknowledgement that conditions such as heart disease may be stress-related, in general, traditional medicine does not consider mind-body techniques to be a vital part of the treatment of the vast majority of medical disorders.

A conscientious holistic practitioner must insure that all available, proven physical treatments are considered. However, complete care of the patient requires that the emotional, psychological and spiritual aspects of the person are also addressed. It is thought that some complementary treatments may in fact be addressing these vital non-physical parts of the whole person and as such are very useful. Often times, western medicine will reject complementary therapies out of hand based on a lack of scientific evidence proving their efficacy. Unfortunately, this bias also results in the rejection of mind-body therapies about which there has been much evidence based research over the last four decades.

Traditional and holistic approaches are based on very different philosophies. People living in western society have been raised to believe that bad things just shouldn't happen. People shouldn't get sick; no one should die, nor even a bad day. If bad things do happen, someone must be responsible (often the doctor), making ours the most litigious society in the world.

A holistic approach embraces a more eastern philosophy which understands that illness, accidents, mistakes and even death are necessary and integral parts of the human existence. No one is to blame; it's just how it is. It is up to each individual to take responsibility for his or her own life, make the necessary changes, and learn to gracefully accept what cannot be changed.

In western culture, illness is viewed only as something horrible which must be gotten rid of; disease is the enemy. The goal of holistic medicine is to decrease the suffering and cure the disease just as it is in western medicine. However, illness can also be viewed as an opportunity to step back and learn something about oneself. Although one would never wish it on himself, illness can be seen as a messenger whose presence, if looked at deeply, can be life transforming. A holistic view comprehends the opportunities for personal growth and healing that illness and yes, even death provides.

Death is another area where traditional and holistic philosophies differ radically. Western doctors and patients alike view death as a failure. When nothing more can be done to cure an illness, the patient may feel abandoned by the doctor who in turn may feel that he or she has failed in some way. Paradoxically, there are also times when people who are nearing the natural end of their lives undergo excruciating, invasive, last-ditch attempts at keeping their bodies alive when death is inevitably imminent. The cost of medical care in the last few days of a person's life is often more than it cost up to that time. The unnecessary suffering that some people withstand before they die is a travesty. But, this doesn't happen because doctors are unfeeling ghouls; this happens because western society demands it; one of the real tragedies of our culture. Thankfully, due to the continuing and heroic efforts of the hospice movement, we are beginning to embrace a more holistic approach to death and dying; that is death with dignity.

In fact, there is much for a practitioner to do at the end of a patient's life. Traditional medicine can and must provide all of the comfort measures available. There may not be a cure, but there is no practice in medicine more important than this. The best gift that a health care practitioner can give, be they medical or holistic, is to provide an environment of compassion and openness that helps ease the patient's transition from this world to whatever comes next. This is a time for the person to tie up loose ends, finish any unfinished business and to evaluate their life before they make their transition. Like it or not, death is the one thing that we all ultimately experience, and thus, it is a vital part of each individual's journey. Think about how much more peaceful a person's death (and life) would be with an attitude of acceptance rather than rejection of this certainty.

Who is responsible for curing illness and healing? Traditional medicine believes the doctor has all the responsibility and all the power. Patients are not assumed to have anything to contribute other than making lifestyle changes that adversely affect their physical bodies, such as smoking cessation, weight loss, and exercise. But when push comes to shove, the first person we want to blame or even file a lawsuit against is the doctor for not curing us, or the tobacco companies for selling us cigarettes. From this perspective, traditional medicine, as good as it is, has a tendency to negate a person's ability power and responsibility to contribute to his or her own healing. This has perpetuated a cultural trend of taking no personal responsibility, wanting magic pills for instant relief and cure, and spending much of our lives either panicking about or avoiding the inevitable - the primary cause of human suffering.

A holistic approach requires that one not only accept personal responsibility to take better care of his/her physical body, but also to have a healthy attitude, and address the psychological and spiritual issues that effect their health. The doctor's responsibility then becomes providing the best physical treatment and technology that western medicine has to offer, the rest is personal responsibility.

So, exactly what does an individual's responsibility for his/her own health entail? Traditional medicine provides the simple answer to that question – good nutrition and physical exercise. No one will dispute that a healthy diet and rejecting toxic influences such as smoking, drugs, and excessive alcohol is in our best interest. Moderation and balance in all things is a simple (but not easy) code to live by. Exercise will undoubtedly prolong one's life, and even more importantly, provide a better quality of life. Nobody claims that this is easy.

But, there is more. For ultimate health and well-being, one must also practice mental self-regulation and have a sense of his or her own spiritual/philosophical values. Mental self-regulation is the concept that we all have it within our power to make conscious choices to develop more positive and loving attitudes such as gratitude, generosity and acceptance. These will not only bring more peace, happiness and equanimity into our lives, but will cause healthful changes in our physiology. In addition, attention to spiritual (not necessarily religious) values like forgiveness, tolerance, charity, love and compassion is the secret of a truly satisfying, full, happy and healthy life. Rarely mentioned within the context of traditional medicine, these things form the basis of a holistic approach to life and health. Although we all will have challenges and tragic situations in our lives that cannot be changed, mental self-regulation means that we can change our minds about them. Changing your mind and attitude in a more positive direction can be done, and it will make you happier. But what you may not realize is that changing your mind also changes your physiologic brain function, which in turn changes your body's physiology.

Meditation is one way to help us to change our minds. It helps us to accept and make peace with that which we cannot change, and connects us to the best, most loving, and incredibly brilliant part of ourselves: our inner being.

Have you ever noticed that some people are intrinsically happy, while others are generally gloomy? Come to find out, these people have different brain physiology. A recent study in the *Journal of Psychosomatic Medicine* shows that meditation actually changes the brain function in gloomy people to be more like the brain function of those who consider themselves happy. In this study, electroencephalograms (EEGs) and positron emission tomography (PET) scans showed that the brain wave patterns in gloomy people are most active in the amygdala (the fear center) of the brain and in the right prefrontal cortex; whereas in happy people, the left prefrontal cortex is the most active area. When gloomy people meditate, however, the activity shifts to the left prefrontal cortex, just as it is in happy people.[1] So clearly, meditation can change a person neurophysiologically from sad to happy.

This is all very nice, but how does it work? What actually happens? How does changing one's mind actually make a difference in a person's health and well-being? How do emotions directly impact the health status of one's body? Read on.

CHAPTER THREE

The Biophysiology of Thought, Emotion and Stress

What is stress? I don't know about you, but for me, just hearing the word makes me grimace and my whole body tightens as if bracing itself for some ominous, invisible shoe to drop. So just the word, though only a verbal representation of something with which we are all too familiar, brings on myriad emotions and physical sensations which are unpleasant at best.

But, stress is not necessarily all bad. Stress level and ability to function fall on a bell-shaped curve. The top of the bell curve represents the optimal amount of stress necessary to perform required tasks most efficiently. One needs a little stress to get up in the morning, get breakfast, get the kids off to school, get ready for work, and make mental preparations for the day. If, however, the stress level increases beyond this point—the kids are fighting, you run out of coffee, you're sitting in a traffic jam and miss your appointment— there is a corresponding decrease in your ability to function and feel well. It is this downward slope of the curve that causes difficulties.

Another useful function of stress is the fight or flight response. The stress response was originally programmed into the primitive homo sapien's brain as physical protection against situations of real danger. Ponder for a moment, what happens physiologically for a cave man to escape from the clutches of a sabre tooth tiger.

In the face of real danger, the brain produces epinephrine, cortisol (a short-term repair hormone), and endorphins. These increase mental arousal and alertness, a capital idea if being chased by something threatening one's life. Heart rate, blood pressure, the force of each heartbeat and even the volume of blood increase to get the necessary oxygen and nutrients to the tissues that need energy for a quick escape. Platelets become sticky so that wounds inflicted by a predator can clot, decreasing the possibility of lethal blood loss after injury. The stress response allows one to react with strong emotions, such as fear and anger, to keep him safe. This is not the time to feel mellow and relaxed. Metabolically, the body increases its formation of glucose and fatty acids for the quick blast of energy it needs for fight and flight.

When confronted with danger, blood rushes to the large muscles, allowing the person to react and run at maximum speed. The muscles contract and tense, particularly the extremities, back, neck, face and jaw. The immune system is also called into action as increased cortisol causes a temporary increase in the immune and inflammatory response. The gastrointestinal tract acts quickly to move recently ingested food through the esophagus by causing forceful esophageal contractions. And there is an increase of gastric acid in the stomach to start the digestive process. Once food is in the stomach and somewhat out of the way, digestion slows down as the blood supply is shifted to the heart and extremities where it is needed the most. Even the reproductive tract is curtailed at this time. It would be unhelpful to be thinking about sex when being chased by a sabre tooth tiger.

Without this very useful stress response, we would not have survived as a species. Fight or flight has been and continues to be a safeguard to our survival. When used as nature intended, no harm comes to our physical bodies because when the threat is over, all systems return to their baseline state of rest.

So, how did we move from this innate adaptive response to the overwhelming levels of stress from which we suffer today? Throughout man's evolution, he has developed a larger cerebral cortex. The downside is that in this advanced brain, even the *perception* of danger elicits exactly the same physiologic response as actual danger. In other words, for the entire biophysiologic fight-flight cascade to take place, all that is required is a person's fear or anxiety about something, real or perceived. A mere fearful thought causes one's body to react as though there was actually a real threat. This response is usually out of proportion to the actual event itself.

Biophysiologic stress happens even when you are not consciously aware of feeling stressed. In contemporary western culture, obsessive busy-ness, production and external demands have become the norm. We race from one activity to the next and are not cognizant of the negative physiologic impact it is having. We recognize stress only as it relates to difficulties in our lives, when in fact unhealthy stress has become a culturally acceptable expense even in what is considered the best of times. We feel that if we are not busy running around doing six things at a time, we won't measure up. Thus, stress has been built into the very fabric of our society. Taking time for ourselves—reading, meditating—is viewed as suspect, making it unlikely that we will take time required for rest and relaxation.

What are some examples of everyday stress? It could be as simple as having to wait in line at the post office, shopping or the bank; having a disagreement with your spouse or needing to speak to your boss about dissatisfaction with your job. Or, God forbid, you run out of coffee in the morning, get stuck in traffic, are put on hold for 15 minutes, or are not able to access the internet. These stressors are of course minor compared to the larger, more pervasive issues of our lives such as relationship problems, raising cantankerous teenagers, illness or death in the family. The list of stressors that we all live with everyday is infinite, as are the possibilities that our bodies will be assaulted again and again by the physiologic stress response that we confront in modern-day life.

So, each time you worry about anything big or small, even if your fear is completely unfounded, or if you have crammed too may responsibilities or activities into your day, your body will increase its metabolism, increase its cardiovascular work, and increase breathing rate and blood flow for which your health will eventually pay a price.

Given this background, it is easy to understand how prolonged or repeated stress can affect our well-being, and why a chronically stressed person will have an increased risk of high blood pressure, abnormal heart rate and rhythm, an increased risk of heart attack, heart failure and stroke. The increased fatty acid production caused by the body's perceived need for increased energy eventually causes damage to blood vessels which supply the heart and peripheral structures by depositing atherosclerotic plaques. And those sticky platelets so important for clotting blood in injury are not so helpful when they are forming clots in the coronary arteries, which can lead to myocardial infarction (heart attack).

Why are chronically stressed people prone to a variety of mood disturbances? Remember, there is an increase in cortisol in times of stress. Though useful in the short term, longer term elevations of cortisol can lead to a decrease in tryptophan which can cause depression. The increased arousal necessary to flee danger can also result in persistent anger, frustration, insomnia and anxiety, which in and of itself further perpetuates physiologic stress changes.

Although short term increases in cortisol help with repair, on going stress can damage our immune system. Over the long term, cortisol is an immunosuppressant, which means its presence prevents the formation of new immune cells and inhibits the ones already present. Cortisol damages natural killer cells whose vital function is seeking out and destroying viruses, bacteria and cancer cells. It also inhibits the T cells ability to fight HIV infection and autoimmune disease. So, although stress may not be the primary cause of infections or cancer, one can see how it could make a person susceptible to these kinds of illnesses.

A stressed gastrointestinal tract may result in increased esophageal contraction, resulting in painful spasm and increased gastric acid, causing ulcer and reflux disease. Abnormalities in motility at the level of the intestines are responsible for the unpredictable appearance of constipation and/or diarrhea, otherwise known as irritable bowel syndrome.

Ongoing stress has been proven to be one of the leading causes of infertility, due to the potentially permanent shutdown of the reproductive tract if stress is unremitting.

Neck and back pain are two of the most common complaints I have treated in my 20-plus years of working as an emergency room physician. Stress is a significant factor in these symptoms. Even in cases of actual physical injury, how long the pain lasts and its intensity directly relates to how much the person worries about it. In fact, prolonged stress not only causes chronic neck and back pain, headaches and muscle spasm, but also will make any pain that a person has anywhere in his or her body worse. When one understands the effects of stress on the musculoskeletal system (a constant tensing of the body's musculature), it is obvious why people who are under a lot of stress will have more pain and why practically everyone has severe neck pain, back pain or headaches at some point in time.

Yet, when the physician suggests that the pain may be stress-related, patients feel as though they are not being taken seriously. To most people, stress–related or what used to be termed, "psychosomatic" illness only happens to crazy people. So, the mere suggestion that this is the cause of one's complaint is tantamount to a patient's feeling as though the doctor considers him or her to be mentally imbalanced. This causes further resistance to looking at what is really going on in the patient's body. Whether the doctor actually makes the statement or not, patients often leave the physician's office with the impression that, the doctor feels these symptoms are "all in my head." This recognition of the mind-body connection is not helpful unless followed up by a detailed explanation of what actually happens to the body as a result of one's thoughts and emotions. Yet, most doctors in the course of their busy day can't take the time to explain all of this. So prescriptions are given to temporarily alleviate the pain; some helpful, some not. But neither the physician nor the patient is addressing the underlying issues.

How is everyday stress actually worse than being chased by a sabre tooth tiger? It is worse because it never goes away. There is never any resolution, as there is when situations of real danger are over. Our bodies get bombarded with a constant physiologic assault, potentially damaging every tissue and cell of the body.

There are hundreds of studies that show how every part of our physiology is affected by stress. Dr. Herbert Benson, a cardiologist from Harvard Medical School, has written several books pertaining to the understanding of the power of the mind-body connection. (See Bibliography.)

Studies have shown that people who have recently lost a partner or spouse will have a decrease in the number of natural killer cells, increasing the likelihood of infection or cancer. Although the death of a spouse causes significant changes in the immune system's ability to function, divorce and separation are even more devastating.[1] But even with less extreme stressful circumstances, there are impressive changes. For example, students show a similar decrease in natural killer cells during exams, thus the increased incidence of upper respiratory illnesses during this time.[2]

Laboratory science has studied the physiologic ramifications of stress on rats. These studies show a decrease in T cell function similar to what happens with humans. The result of this assault on the animals' immune system is an increase in infections and tumor growth. Chronically stressed rats have also been shown to have enlarged adrenal glands from the ongoing production of cortisol and burnt out thymus glands (where T cells are made).[3]

So, in a society where stress is the expected norm, it follows that one must carry on silently, never giving voice to the ongoing exhaustion and frustration. It is not acceptable for us to constantly blow off steam, so most of us deal with stress by internalizing it. As a result, we remain angry, resentful and depressed. We have no physiologic release or resolution, so stress continues to wreak its biophysiologic havoc, even though the inciting incident may be long gone.

Still not convinced? Have you ever had headaches, neck or back pain, racing heart, dry mouth, sweaty palms, indigestion, irritable bowel syndrome, jaw pain, persistent fatigue, dizziness or difficulty sleeping? Have you ever gone through periods when you are sad, weepy, easily upset, ready to explode, or unhappy for no apparent reason? Do you ever feel compelled to eat more junk food, drink more alcohol and smoke more cigarettes than usual? Are there times when you are more critical, bossier and harder on yourself; more confused, forgetful, spacey, unable to make decisions, and out of control with constant worry? Are there times when life doesn't seem to have any meaning, you feel empty, you lack self-confidence or you become more cynical? Have you ever gone through periods when your relationships are not satisfying, you are grumpy, intolerant, have a decreased sex drive and a need to isolate yourself from interaction with others? If any of these things are true at one time or another, stress is the number one cause. All this gives new meaning to that unfortunate sentiment, "it's all in your head."

Now you can understand that, although much of our suffering is precipitated by our thoughts and worries, even though we may not always be aware of them, there are irrefutable physical ramifications. And yes, you do become physically ill and your physical pain and suffering are real. The deal with stress is, if you can't control it, it will control you and your body.

Thankfully, there are many traditional treatments for what stress does to us. Although this is a book about how you can help yourself, *do not* neglect what western medicine has to offer. Pharmaceuticals including anti-hypertensive, anti-depressant, anti-inflammatory, cardiac medications, antacids, H2 blockers, chemotherapeutic agents, and antibiotics are godsends. Despite a regular meditation practice, I take some of these medicines myself. If you need bypass surgery, infertility, or GI procedures, by all means, have them done. Chanting and meditation are no substitutes for an appendectomy (though it might be interesting to try it while waiting for the doctor in the ER!). For psychological or emotional distress, psychotherapy and psychoactive medications must be considered.

Despite popular skepticism held by some medical traditionalists, complementary therapies including mind-body medicine, massage, acupuncture, Reiki, aromatherapy, and chiropractic treatments can be helpful, as it is likely that they may be treating the emotional, psychological and spiritual symptoms not easily amenable to the rigors of materialistic science. But taking into consideration the effects of stress, even if they do nothing more than help the patient relax, they would have accomplished a great deal. I am reminded of the words of Dr. Rudolf Virchow, "Absence of proof does not necessarily mean proof of absence." Having said that, I applaud and welcome the efforts on the part of these practitioners to continue their good work and do the studies that are required for scientific credibility.

Mind-Body medicine is the area of complementary medicine that has been the most extensively studied and its value proven again and again. Mind-body practices, including relaxation techniques, meditation, exercise, proper nutrition, cognitive therapies, martial arts (yoga, tai chi), and spiritual practices all help to make your body a less desirable host for illness and discomfort, and will likely make you a happier, more balanced individual.

Just taking occasional moments to stop and attend to your breathing makes a huge difference in both your perceived and physiologic stress. Dr. Bernie Siegel refers to these restful moments each day as "healing intervals." Conscious breathing, meditation, exercise, walking on the beach, prayer, and reading are some of my personal healing intervals. They do not have to be many; and they do not have to take a long time. You can benefit from just stopping and becoming consciously aware of yourself and your needs. Quiet healing intervals help you to see that, even during times of intolerable stress, the person inside—the real you—is doing fine and will get through these challenges.

"Stress hardiness" describes those people who seem the best able to cope with stressful situations in their lives. Studies have been done which attempt to understand those personality traits that make a person "stress hardy." Susan Kobasa, 1979, looked at how people dealt with losing their jobs as their workplace was being restructured. They discovered that those who coped well upon losing their jobs were people who tended to look at change as a challenge rather than as a stressor. Job loss was seen as an opportunity to explore other interests; positive meaning was found in what could have been a devastating situation.

These people seem to understand that, although there are situations in their lives over which they have no control, they know that they can control their minds' reaction to them; and that makes all the difference. They have a sense of commitment to whatever they do and understand at a deep level what the Buddhists have been teaching for centuries; that suffering is inevitable, but that misery (our negative reaction to suffering) is optional and totally dependent upon our thoughts and attitudes.[4]

Avoiding perfectionism is another way to decrease stress. We are so hard on ourselves and our society is hard on us. We are fallible humans who can't give ourselves a break. We do our bodies and ourselves a disservice by our relentless desire to be better, thinner, smarter, and more successful. It is tragic when you don't realize that the real you, the person that you will come to know during meditative periods of silence, is perfect just as you are. This program will have been hugely successful if you learn nothing more than this.

Laughter, by itself an effective stress reducer, has been shown to assist the body's attempt at healing. Norman Cousins and Loretta LaRoche have written wonderful, entertaining, intelligent books, and have lectured on this topic. Even western medicine is beginning to appreciate and study the physiologic effects of laughter. A recent study entitled, "Neuroendocrine and Stress Hormone Changes during Mirthful Laughter," done at Loma Linda University and published by the *American Journal of Medical Science*, measured stress hormone levels and showed that, "Mirthful laughter experience appears to decrease levels of serum cortisol, epinephrine and growth hormone. These biochemical changes have implications for the reversal of the neuroendocrine and classical stress hormone response."[5] Translation... laughter is good for decreasing the effect that stress has on your body. Western science has a way of making even the subject of laughter intense. It is clear to me why my brow was deeply furrowed and I had headaches all through medical school.

There is evidence that emotions, even if they are an act, have significant physical impact on the body. Paul Ekman, at the University of California, San Francisco, asked people to force their faces into smiles. They not only felt happier, but also had measurable neurologic and physiolologic changes consistent with relaxation. Those who forced their faces into expressions of fear or sadness had measurable increases in stress chemicals.[6] Immunologist, Nicholas Hall, studied actors and learned that those in comedies and upbeat productions had long lasting increases in immune function while those in serious or tragic productions had a corresponding decrease in measurable immune indicators. These studies suggest that we can make conscious decisions to change our moods and emotions and that our physiology will change accordingly.

Psychneuroimmunology is a relatively new field that looks specifically at how thoughts and emotions affect the physical body. Dr. Candace Pert first discovered that humans make mood enhancing endorphins and enkephalins in response to exercise. She and others have gone on to discover that "neuropeptides" are formed in our bodies every time we have a thought. In fact, our bodies can be thought of as having our very own little pharmacies in which every kind of drug you can imagine is manufactured in response to what we are thinking. Studies have shown that a person who is feeling peaceful and tranquil is actually making a substance that closely resembles valium. Anxious persons, as we already know, make cortisol and epinephrine; and people who are excited or exhilarated actually make interferon-like substances, which are potent anti-cancer agents. Just imagine the difference it would make for people to comprehend the power of a conscious decision to change their minds!

What about placebos? Why is it that people can be given sugar pills for a variety of illnesses and get better even though the sugar pill has no actual effect on the disease process? We assume that anyone who would fall for the old placebo trick must just be neurotic or otherwise emotionally unstable. In fact, what actually appears to happen is that just the thought that a placebo pill is really an antibiotic, tranquilizer, anti-cancer drug or any drug imaginable is stimulus enough for the brain to initiate manufacturing just the drug that we need! If you add to that the actual pharmacologic action of the medicine that your doctor gives you, you benefit from both the action of the drug and the drugs made in your own bio-pharmacy in response to your beliefs and thoughts.

So, are you beginning to understand how important your beliefs are in your own healing process? Doctors are helpful and necessary; but your participation is also crucial. Unfortunately, my friend Lynn was never given this message, making her treatment less useful than it might have been. By not engaging her in her own healing process, she became dis-empowered. The damage done to her spirit as a result was even worse than the inability of western medicine to cure her body.

Something known as the nocebo effect is also worthy of mention here. It has been found that if a doctor tells a patient that he/she has six months to live, that person is likely to live for exactly six months. If you are told that, "you will have this [disease/ailment] for the rest of your life," there is a good chance that you will in fact suffer from that ailment for the rest of your life. What our doctors say to us is more powerful than you can imagine. In fact, doctors don't usually like to make these statements, but often do only if the patient insists. Remember, you are not a statistic; everyone heals in his/her own unique way. Never allow such statements to become self-fulfilling prophesies. Just consider that any information you get is only a small part of the whole. Then put all your energy into securing whatever is the best possible outcome for yourself.

Mind-Body medicine is the discipline that uses the amazing power of our minds to cure or assist traditional medicine in curing physical illness; and more importantly, to heal you emotionally, psychologically and spiritually. Rachel Naomi Remen said, "Not everyone can be cured, but everyone can be healed. Healing is all about finding peace in yourself." If I had to choose, I'd go for the healing. So, although your doctor is the "go to" person for a cure, a loved one, a compassionate nurse, your golden retriever or anyone who shows you love and kindness can help to heal you. But most of all, healing can be done silently by and for yourself.

Over the last three decades, hundreds of studies have been done showing the impact of mind-body practices on our physical bodies. Herb Benson and others have reported that meditating 20 minutes, twice a day, will drop blood pressure, on the average, by seven points systolic and four points diastolic. This is approximately equal to the effect of a single blood pressure medication and without side effects. If yoga is added, blood pressure drops on the average by 20 systolic and 14 diastolic, [7] roughly equal to using two anti-hypertensive agents.

A person's spiritual and/or religious beliefs can also have a significant impact on his or her health and well-being. Prayer, like meditation, is a potent mind-body practice. Researchers have learned that people who attend regular religious services, or have a regular prayer or meditation practice will have a 40 percent less chance of developing hypertension[8] and a 20 percent decrease in hospital stay after heart surgery[9]. Religious or spiritually inclined HIV patients have higher CD4 counts[10]. And women with hip fractures who pray regularly are able to walk longer distances at the time of their hospital discharge.[11]

Buddhist meditation practitioners have been shown to have lower cortisol levels, higher serum protein levels (a gross measure of nutritional status), lower blood pressure, lower heart rate and better lung function than non-meditating controls.[12] In fact, there have been many studies showing that transcendental meditation reverses stress related illness, makes people healthier, and reduces medical costs as much as 13 percent per year. The improvement in health is most significant for older age groups and people with the worst overall health. Hospitalizations for cancer are 55 percent lower in those people who meditate on a regular basis.

In Holland, those who practice transcendental meditation get a 30 percent discount in health insurance due to fewer hospital admissions and decreases in every type of illness or physical complaint. And a large smoking cessation study has shown that people who meditate 20 minutes, twice a day will have an 80 percent success rate as compared to those who do not meditate, whose chance of success is approximately 5 percent.[13]

So, one might ask, why isn't Mind-Body medicine more mainstream? Herbert Benson, M.D. one of the contemporary mind-body medicine gurus has dedicated his career doing impressive, exquisite scientific inquiry on the power of the mind to influence the body. Although no one would dispute his genius, traditional western medicine is a tough nut to crack.

Dr. Benson was at Harvard during the days of Timothy Leary and Richard Alpert (Ram Dass). He became intrigued when some of these LSD experimenters went to India in search of answers to their questions about the real nature of consciousness. What fascinated him was his observation that when these people returned from India, they were calmer and had peaceful attitudes. For some reason they had lower baseline blood pressure and heart rates. Overall, they appeared to be super healthy beings. After many years of study, Dr. Benson determined that it was their meditation practice that made them so different.

Something happens in meditation that changes the individual physiologically. These observations were what lead up to what Dr. Benson has termed the "relaxation response." The relaxation response has effects that are the exact opposite and in fact counteract the effects of the fight or flight response. When one elicits this response, he achieves a deep state of rest in which heart rate, blood pressure, breathing, and metabolic rate, gastric acid production, and muscle tension all decrease. There is also an improvement of mood, coping ability, immune function and fertility.

Elicitation of the relaxation response, Dr. Benson learned, is simple and boils down to two steps, "the repetition of a word, sound, prayer or muscular activity with a passive return to the repetition when other thoughts intrude."[14] The repetition of mantras, such as 'om' forms the basis of transcendental meditation, but any word or phrase that has meaning for the person using it works just as well. The words, "love", "peace," the name of someone you love or phrases such as,

"Thy will be done" or "Hail Mary full of Grace," have the same effect.

One of Dr. Benson's most impressive findings is that if one meditates (essentially eliciting the relaxation response) for 20 minutes twice each day, every measurable stress indicator is effectively blunted, not only while meditating, but for a 24-hour period, [15] an incredible finding, don't you think?

Jon Kabat-Zinn, Professor of Medicine Emeritus and founding director of the stress reduction clinic and Center for Mindfulness at the University of Massachusetts Medical Center has further shown that this phenomenon is not due to the placebo effect. He studied a group of people who didn't believe that meditation actually did anything. He taught them a simple meditation practice and instructed them to meditate 20 minutes, twice a day. What he found was that, even people who did not believe that meditating would make any difference, had changes that were measurable and reproducible.[16] Kabat-Zinn says, "Like Penicillin, this will work whether you believe it or not" and "You don't have to like it, you just have to do it."[17]

Meditation Practice: Transcendental Meditation, Relaxation Response

Close this book; close your eyes. Focus first on your breathing, then chose a word or phrase that is meaningful to you and say it quietly to yourself on each in-breath or each out-breath. Each time your mind wanders, which it will, just bring it back to your chosen repetition. Please take five minutes now for this exercise.

This simple exercise is the basis of every meditative practice. You need learn nothing more to start living a life that is less damaged by stress. Take a moment to notice how, in this short exercise, your breathing slowed down and your body felt more calm and relaxed. Did you sense that even though your thoughts were still present, they seemed more distant? And as you breathed and focused, did you get a sense that there is a silent being residing in your body who quietly witnesses everything? If not, you will by the end of this book and audio meditations.

Meditation is only one of the many ways of eliciting the relaxation response. Progressive muscle relaxation, yoga, tai chi, repetitive physical exercise, prayer from any religious tradition, and music, when listened to with focus, have similar physiologic effects. The key word here is *focus,* which will be discussed in detail in later chapters.

As a traditional physician, I must mention a few caveats to all complementary or alternative practices. First, in a quote whose original author is unknown, "Keep an open mind, but don't let your brain fall out." Make sure that you cover all the scientifically proven bases regarding your health while pursuing any alternatives. Remember, western medicine has almost single handedly increased the human lifespan from three to up to eight decades over the last few hundred years; they really are the "cure guys." Be cautious of any treatment or practitioner who discourages you from obtaining conventional medical care or may interact with it in a dangerous way.

I also ask you to be aware of something called "new age fascism." One can get the impression that anyone who is positive enough, uses the right affirmations, and practices daily meditation, will be guaranteed a cure; and that failure to achieve this end is somehow that person's fault. It is even more disturbing when people actually blame themselves for getting cancer or some other illness. Sadly, many people, including my friend Lynn, have gone down this slippery slope. This was not only detrimental to her purpose of getting better but is pure **NONSENSE.** Sure, we could all make more healthy decisions in our lives, but that is part of what makes us human. There is no place here for guilt. Taking on guilt is the unhealthiest decision you can make for yourself.

Meditation and other mind-body practices give your health the best possible shot by giving your inner being the opportunity to help cure you physically and heal you on a much deeper and frankly more important level.

CHAPTER FOUR

Meditation

Meditation cannot be taught until one understands the value of solitude. The concept of spending time by oneself is something that runs counter to our societal norm. For many, being alone is not only undesirable; it is something to be avoided at all cost. Although less taboo than it was 30 years ago, there is still a sense that one must be a part of a couple, or at the very least, always be in the presence of other people. Going to the movies, out to dinner or on a trip alone is unusual and fraught with terror for many. How many people stay in intolerable marriages solely out of the fear of being alone?

The whole point of meditation is to become familiar with one's own inner being. This cannot be done with anyone but yourself. So a commitment to spending time in solitude is a must. Our loved ones can help us in many ways; and though we treasure their presence in our lives, we can only get to know our true selves and recharge our spirits when we are alone and in silence.

So, what exactly is meditation? Meditation is a period of time in which you consciously stop all activities and thought patterns, and spend that time in intense focus. What does meditation do? Meditation quiets the conscious mind, known also as the left brain or ego. The ego is the business part of our being that tends to the important motions of everyday life—planning, scheming, worrying, criticizing and doing. This is also the fearful, critical and judgmental part of us, but a part without which we could not function as human beings. Generally caught up in thoughts of the past or the future, the ego has little time to spend enjoying or even noticing the present. MRI and PET scans of the brain have shown that the amygdala, the part of the brain responsible for fear, anger, avoidance and defensiveness, shuts down during meditation, and becomes activated during stress.[1] Though it is a vital structure in the limbic system; it is nice to get a break from one's amygdala from time to time.

With the left brain's business temporarily anesthetized, the generally silent right brain, also known as the true, higher, spiritual self, or Buddha nature, has a chance to express itself. The right brain is the home of our inner wisdom, emotions, creativity, compassion, unconditional love, generosity, inspiration and is our connection to our spirituality. In our day-to-day lives, we spend the vast majority of our time in left-brain endeavors. Look at what we are missing out on as a result. Imagine for a moment what a different place the world would be if we all spent even 10 percent of our energy in right brain pursuits!

Buddhists believe that everyone has a brilliant and all-loving inner space to which meditation provides access. The goal of all Buddhist meditation practices is to help us to live our lives more in sync with what they refer to as our Buddha nature. This differs little from the Christian concept of prayer bringing one closer to one's soul. In fact, many religious traditions believe that there is something of a Divine nature within each one of us, and that prayer and meditation can access that divinity and use it for our greater good.

Meditation can also have an effect on beings outside of ourselves. Dr. Herb Benson tells the story of a friend of his who was meditating beside a lake, as was her usual practice. One day, there were two very noisy swans squabbling some distance away from her. As she concentrated on her breathing, she let this noise drift away. After a little while, she noticed that the noise had stopped and that the swans were slowly drifting toward her. Continuing to meditate, she soon felt a presence near her and sure enough, the swans were now on the shore by her feet. After a few more minutes of silence, she felt the neck of one swan drape itself across her lap and a moment later, the other did the same on the opposite side. Improbable as this may seem, I have noticed the same thing happen to my dogs when I meditate. I have even attracted the attention of random dogs who occasionally appear and lay down next to me while I'm meditating on the beach. There is no doubt in my mind that meditation and prayer have far reaching effects extending beyond the human realm.

Despite positive effects on our bodies and on others, it is important not to have preordained goals and to meditate solely for the sake of meditation. This is a time when your inner being has a chance to speak to you. When your left-brain is in the forefront, your ego is trying to tell your inner wisdom what to do and this defeats the whole purpose. So despite the potential for decreases in blood pressure, chronic pain, headaches, irritable bowel syndrome, and other ailments, it is best to consider these as desirable "side effects" of a practice which is valuable even if none of these things happen.

Another benefit of meditation is the likelihood that your relationships will improve. In meditation, you spend more time with the best, most loving part of your inner self. This can impact your relationships in positive ways. And your ability to concentrate improves as, during meditation, you bring your mind back to its focus repeatedly. As with everything else, practice makes perfect.

Another benefit of meditation is its ability to help you heal. According to Mark Barasch, author of several books on healing and former editor in chief of the *New Age Journal,* "Healing implies restoration of communication with ourselves. If we're present to ourselves, our body's wisdom will let us know what we need." Remember that healing can take place even without a physical cure. Healing is all about finding inner peace and the only one who can bring you peace is yourself. If you take any part of this book and integrate it into your daily life, your life will change for the better. Meditation is a gift that you give yourself.

The mystical guru image that most westerners have of those who meditate discourages many from starting their own practice. Although sitting in full lotus for hours at a time with an empty mind may be out of reach for most of us, this is only one of many possible practices. Mindfulness, lovingkindness, Tonglen, contemplation, transcendental meditation, imagery and prayer are just a few of the formal sitting meditation practices. Yoga, tai chi, stretching, walking, aerobics or any exercise done *with focus* can be meditation in motion. In fact, anything you do can be turned into a meditation if done with focus. Meditation is individual; you can make it up as you go.

Even music, when used as your meditative focus, can be a powerful meditation. Paying attention to each note, letting the music take you where it will, or focusing on inspiring lyrics is a type of meditation with many of the same healthful side effects. A recent study has shown that listening to music can change one's biophysiology. Narcan, a medication used in hospitals when a person is suspected of having a drug overdose, works by reversing the action of the suspected drug. Interestingly, Narcan also appears to decrease ones enjoyment of music, suggesting that music is just one more stimulus for turning on a person's inner pharmacy to make euphoric substances in our bodies.

As helpful as this may be, some of you may be thinking, "I don't have time to meditate". But when you find yourself waiting in line, stuck in traffic, pumping gas, or exercising, stop, breathe, focus, and you are meditating. I am not suggesting that you plunk yourself down in the grocery store line looking like some kind of weirdo in some odd posture, but it may be more useful to stop frothing at the mouth and pay attention to your breathing instead.

My favorite time to meditate is when I'm feeling aggravated, like when I am in a hurry and the person ahead of me at the supermarket is arguing over the price of lettuce. At times like these, a useful mantra is, "I could choose peace." Remember, no matter what is happening, **you can always choose peace**. Sometimes you won't want to choose peace and that is perfectly all right. What's important is that your choices are conscious. If you know you have options, you don't have to become a victim of automatic negative responses that pull you into a negative, downward spiral.

I recommend taking a little time to make a list of all the times during the day that you are wasting or are involved in activities that don't add anything of value to your life. Meditation is a far more useful alternative to watching TV, boredom eating, wandering aimlessly at the mall or feeling aggravated. I must confess with some embarrassment that I was able to come up with five hours a week after my children stopped collecting Beanie Babies. Yes, I was one of those crazed individuals who searched high and low for the supposed rare mini plush toys, spending ridiculous amounts of precious time on something providing no real value to anyone (unless you consider the 10 or so crates now in my attic a boon to society). I gained another five hours by relinquishing my obsessive need to watch the conveniently recorded *All My Children* everyday. No offense intended, but in truth, I came to realize that Erica Kane's trials and tribulations, though entertaining, were adding nothing to my spiritual journey.

Meditation can make you more efficient, organized, focused and calm. Studies have shown that meditation may even make you live longer. So now, I don't have time *not* to meditate.

Yogic tradition makes a distinction between yogic age and

chronological age. Chronological age, in this way of thinking, has no meaning, as one is not considered to be alive until he/she has a meditation practice. In my own experience, truer words were never spoken.

So where do you begin? You begin with three words: *Breath, Focus*, and *Relax*. Diaphragmatic or "belly breathing" by itself even without any other focus has been shown to decrease blood pressure and heart rate along with all the other benefits of the relaxation response as previously described. A few moments of deep, conscious breathing, several times a day, will make you more peaceful and relaxed, as well as energized, more efficient and creative. Jon Kabat-Zinn says, "Diaphragmatic breathing represents a mental gearshift that helps you stop spinning your wheels and engaging into the power of your mind. This gets you into your meditative mind."[2]

Meditation Practice: Diaphragmatic Breathing

Take in a gentle but full breath. Instead of shallowly filling your lungs, causing only your chest to rise, have that breath expand your abdomen as well. Spend a few moments with your hand on your abdomen feeling the gentle rising and falling with inspiration and expiration. When you notice that your mind is wandering, simply return to the breathing focus.

Throughout this book, I will provide opportunities for you to practice what I am teaching by means of audio guided meditations. Guided meditations are a great way to get started in your meditation practice, as the words provide the focus needed for the meditative state. Though an intellectual (left brain) understanding of the material can be achieved by reading, engaging the right brain through meditation allows the concepts to be experienced on a deep emotional level as well.

Unlike traditional eastern meditation, I chose to use background music in the audio meditations for several reasons. First, it provides a focus for the beginner. Second, music has potent biopharmacologic effects of its own. And finally, after meditating to certain music for a period of time, you will discover that just hearing the music alone will initiate many of the same physiologic changes enjoyed with meditation.

As you become more experienced and comfortable with your own practice, you will no longer need to be guided through your meditation. However, each time you go back to them you will understand them on a deeper level.

Please take a few moments to listen to the following recorded meditation:

Basic Meditation Instruction[3]
CD 1, Track 1
Music licensed through Megatrax Production Music, Inc.

Although spending several hours a day meditating is a wonderful thing, the fact is in our everyday lives, it isn't always possible. But if you ever do have the chance to attend a meditation retreat; your meditation will be deeper. The more you do it, the more it does for you. The important thing is that you spend whatever time you can during your day taking a few breaths and spending some time in silence. Lama Surya Das, an American Buddhist Lama, says that "several mini meditations each day are significantly better than one longy."[4]

A short meditation can be as simple as stopping and focusing on the breath, or counting slowly to 10 with each out breath. Or you can focus on counting 1, 2, 3, 4 on the in breath and 4, 3, 2, 1 on the out breath. Another method is to focus on the pauses between each in breath and out breath. This pause is a great place to experience your own silence.

Progressive muscle relaxation or a body scan is an effective way to get into a meditative state and provides the basis for most other meditation practices. It is vital that one pays attention to how his/her body is feeling as physical symptoms may be there to get us to attend to imbalance in our lives. James Joyce wrote in his book, *A Painful Case,* that the main character Mr. Duffy "lived a short distance from his body." When you think about it, we all live a short distance from our bodies. Think of the number of times each day that we ignore hunger, tight muscles, or even the fact that we need to use the bathroom because we are too busy.

A person can't expect to heal himself without tuning in to listen to his body's wisdom. Progressive muscle relaxation is a method in which you consciously tense and relax the various muscles of your body. This exercise not only relaxes you, but it makes you more aware of how tension in your muscles feels. With this increased awareness, you will be more likely to tend to these sensations during times of stress. The sooner you pay attention to what stress is doing to your body, the sooner you can address it.

Progressive Muscle Relaxation[5]
CD 1, Track 2
Music licensed through Megatrax Production Music, Inc.

The body scan is a shortened form of progressive muscle relaxation in which you start from the head down or the feet up and attend to how every part of your body is feeling. This is done without conscious tensing and relaxing the muscles as in progressive muscle relaxation. This focus not only gets you into a deeper meditative state, but it is gives your body the message that you really do care about yourself and that you are paying attention.

If you are considering a meditation practice, here are a few practical tips. It is ideal if you have a regular schedule for meditating. First thing in the morning is great if you can get out of bed a little earlier. Meditation is restful and is probably better for you than that extra hour of sleep. If you have a busy schedule with limited time in your day, frequent "mini" meditations can be done any time throughout the day. If you are a student, close your eyes and breathe for 10 minutes before each test and study session. One hour of relaxed studying will be more productive then several hours of spastic, frantic studying. And your test taking ability will sky-rocket if you are relaxed and allowing your right brain to contribute its wisdom. A few minutes of quiet focus, especially before stressful meetings, presentations or anxiety-provoking human encounters will allow you to enter each situation in a more relaxed, conscious way making each task of the day more productive and satisfying.

Don't be too hard on yourself and worry about getting it "right." The only way you cannot do it right, is not to do it. Try not to have expectations; just be with whatever comes up and accept whatever is. If your left brain interferes with mind chatter, close your eyes, breathe, and let the thoughts drift into the background. Expectations are a left brain phenomenon and can be temporarily put to rest.

Exercising before meditation can give you a head start into getting into the meditative mind, as it encourages your body's awareness, decreases stress hormones and increases brain alpha wave activity. Meditation further increases this relaxed alpha state

Most of us have heard the saying, "Don't just sit there, do something." When it comes to meditating, however, the statement needs be, "Don't just do something, sit there." Just being is the goal; doing needs to be put aside.

Choose a specific location that is only for your meditation practice. My favorite spot is a beach just 10 minutes from my home. Being in nature enhances your meditation; but I also recommend an indoor alternative, as you don't want cold temperatures or inclement weather to discourage your practice. And remember, you can and should meditate any time, anywhere - whenever you have a spare or otherwise wasted moment.

What type of meditation is right for you? In this book, you will be given the opportunity to sample various disciplines. But when all is said and done, whatever meditation you do will be right for you as long as you do it.

Will meditation change your life? Meditation will not make your problems go away or cure your illnesses, nor will it get you off of this planet alive. But it will help you accept and deal with the unavoidable problems of life with some measure of grace, effectively changing the way you look at things. Seeing the world through your right brain makes you aware that, even though on the surface your life may be like the ocean in a hurricane, underneath you are a tranquil, motionless lagoon. An otherwise dreary, drab landscape takes on more color and texture; much like Dorothy entering Oz, you realize that you are not in Kansas anymore; and your experiences become more serene and rich. Like the yogis, in many ways your real life will start with your meditation practice.

Even though I will be teaching Buddhist philosophy in this book, I am not trying to convert you to Buddhism! A philosophy more than a religion, Buddhism teaches intelligent, practical ways to deal with the imperfect reality of human life. The Dalai Lama says, "Be a good Christian, be a good Jew, but use Buddhist meditation techniques to enhance your own life and your own spirituality." Buddhist inspired philosophy and meditation helps you to be the best and most authentic you that you can be, and there is nothing better than that.

Buddhism teaches that life is suffering. Though this may sound depressing, it is actually a realistic view of the nature of our human existence. We all have difficulties, illness, and we ultimately die. We suffer because of our expectation that this is not the way it should be. Buddhism teaches that the way out of suffering is to learn to deal with the inevitable problems of life with grace. Suffering is inevitable, misery is optional; meditation decreases the misery.

Woody Allen's says, "More than any time in history mankind faces a crossroads. One path leads to despair and utter hopelessness, the other, to total extinction. Let us pray we have the wisdom to choose correctly."[6] The good news is we have a way out of this morass, and that way leads directly to our inner being where it all makes sense. Meditation simply helps you to make peace with what is... that is grace.

CHAPTER FIVE

Gratitude

There is no other attitude as worthy of cultivation as gratitude. Taking the time each day to look at all the things you have to be grateful for can't help but make you see your life in an entirely different light. Even during difficult times, there are always beautiful sunsets. If you are reading this book, I can safely assume that you have plenty to eat. There are people who love and care for you. There are blue skies, an almost 100 percent guarantee that the sun will rise every morning. Turning the knob on your radio or iPod will produce music that you enjoy. Our lives are packed full of an infinite number of wonderful things. Unfortunately, we sometimes allow these things to become blanketed in the morass of human difficulties and dilemmas. Feeling gratitude in no way ignores adversity; it just puts it into a larger perspective.

The Irish have many wonderful sayings, "They are not poor that have little, but they who desire much." And, "The richest man, whatever his lot, is the one who's content with whatever he's got." And my personal favorite, "Better a louse in the pot than no meat at all,"[1] humorously making the point that even in the most extreme circumstances, one can be either happy or sad depending on nothing more than how one chooses to interpret his reality.

Gratitude can be a conscious choice, not just a reaction that takes place spontaneously only when something wonderful happens. One must take the time to focus on thanks-giving. Thus, gratitude becomes a meditation unto itself to be done daily by itself or in combination with the rest of your meditation practice.

Writing in a journal a few moments each day, listing the things that gave you joy can change your perspective. Studies have shown the benefit of this practice. In one study, one third of the participants were asked to write about five events that affected them each day, one third to write about five stressful situations, and the final third were asked to write about five things for which they were grateful. After 10 weeks, the gratitude group was more energetic, optimistic and alert, spent more time exercising and taking care of their well-being, had fewer physical complaints and was more altruistic than in either of the other groups.[2] Michael McCullough, from Southern Methodist University, measured gratefulness as a personality trait, and found that people who have this tendency are much more likely to volunteer their time, donate to charities and place less importance on the acquisition of material goods. In fact, it seems that grateful individuals may actually live longer.[3] A grateful person uses adversity as an opportunity to learn more compassion for others.

Holistically speaking, conscious gratefulness is a method of mental self-regulation whose advantages are limitless both for the individual and for everyone he touches. Gratitude turns into loving actions that can't help but benefit the world. Each day as a regular part of your meditation practice or even as a mini meditation while pumping gas or sitting in traffic, close your eyes and visualize your own gratitude slide show of images of whatever good things come into your mind. There are an infinite number of wonderful things about our human existence; a few quick mental images shouldn't be difficult and can make an enormous difference in how you view your life.

Gratitude[4]
CD 1, Track 3
Excerpts from *Words of Gratitude*, Robert A. Emmons and Joanna Hill
Music licensed through Megatrax Production Music, Inc.

CHAPTER SIX

Mindfulness

Mindfulness, one of many Buddhist-inspired forms of meditation, is the practice of having a conscious awareness of everything that exists in the present moment. Mindfulness is a philosophy that teaches that living our lives mindfully, right here and right now is the secret to having the most fulfilling life possible. The regular practice of mindfulness meditation, as with any type of practice, makes us better at living consciously, thereby enriching our lives.

One week before I taught this lecture for the first time, I had the delightful opportunity of taking my younger daughter, Sarah, to Disney World. What struck me was that this particular vacation spot is that it is the very essence of what mindfulness is all about. There is so much going on and so many sensory delights; one doesn't obsess about the past or worry about the future. Each ride, each exhibit, the smells, tastes and sensations of the place just rivet you in present time, which is why I believe it is such an incredibly popular destination. One can't help but become a child again, children being the undisputed masters of mindful awareness. Having the opportunity to spend this time alone with my daughter made it even more mindfully special, as my attention and focus were on her and her alone, making this the best quality time we have ever spent together.

Thich Nhat Hanh, a Vietnamese Buddhist monk and prolific writer/poet, in his book, *The Miracle of Mindfulness,* writes, "Mindfulness itself is the life of awareness, the presence of mindfulness means the presence of life. Mindfulness frees us of forgetfulness and dispersion and makes it possible to live fully each minute, each minute of life. Mindfulness enables us to live."[1] To be mindful is to be aware of every aspect of life, one's feelings, and one's physical sensations of those around you and what you are doing every minute. It's a celebration of the present moment as being vital in life. To practice mindfulness is to be at one with the moment—to fully immerse yourself in whatever is happening moment to moment.

A journal entry I wrote years ago illustrates a few moments of informal mindfulness meditation. During these introspective times, I recognized that paying attention to the details of life was not only relaxing but it had a way of bringing me closer to that soft, sensitive, silent, content part within me

Informal Mindfulness Meditation

While lying on the beach on a hot summer's day, feel the warmth of the sun's rays beating down on your body. Experience the tingling and the slight burning sensation. Enjoy the comfort that the warmth brings. Feel the sand beneath you, the light tickling as you let it trickle through your fingers. Notice the heat the top sand conveys to your feet, and the coolness as you push them underneath. Smell the freshness of the salt air, notice the ocean mist, the cool sea breeze contrasted to the sun's heat.

Become aware of your own breathing; inhale and exhale, deeply and slowly. Enjoy the freshness of the air around. Appreciate your body for how wonderful it can feel. Experience what this total relaxation feels like. Tend to all the sensations your body feels, this is relaxation. Remember it. Treasure it. Open your eyes to the bright blue sky, the fluffy, white, whipped cream clouds. Enjoy the contrasting colors of the sky and the darker blue ocean. Notice the constantly changing hues and shades of the water – the greenish tinge over the sandbar, the ink-blue over the ocean's depths. Breathe in and breathe out, experience your life as your life as never before.

Be thankful for this moment. Watch little

children stomping fearlessly through the waves, building and smashing sandcastles, running along and diving suddenly down. Splashing, yelling, laughing – experience them for they are a part of this moment. Hear the person breathing beside you; hear the radio on the neighboring blanket. Savor every sensation and observation for itself. Comprehend how it adds to make a beautiful whole, and on and on.

Every singular experience of a person's life can be made much more real, more alive by this kind of careful attention. The relaxation it will bring will be quite a surprise for those who have never experienced it. OK, you might say, this is fine for vacation, but what about every day of my life when there's so much to do? It is especially during these times that the practice of mindfulness – of being fully awake and involved in the present is of utmost importance. Household chores need not be drudgery if they are experienced in their own right. If we look at these jobs only as necessary evils that must be rushed through to get on to some future task, it will be drudgery. The present moment is lost to some future goal which in turn is lost to the one that follows. The net result is a wishing away of your own very special life. This attitude of always looking to the future, rampant in western culture, deprives one of actually living life to its fullest.

Sometime, while washing curtains, attend to that and that alone. Realize that this moment is a part of your life as is any other. Smell the fragrance of the detergent. Feel the soap squishing through your fingers. Watch the wash water become muddy and marvel that so much dirt just wasn't visible while they were up. Watch them become white and soft. Hang them out in the fresh air. Smell how fresh they are. Watch the sun sparkle through them and see the rainbow as the light filters through the wet delicate cloth. Appreciate how quickly the wind dries them, without any assistance from you. Feel the breeze, feel the coolness. Watch the wrinkles disappear as they dry, wonder how that happens.

Notice when they are all dry, take them off the line and feel how soft they are in your arms. Feel the warmth of the iron. Hear the spitting noise of the steam. Notice how easily the iron glides over the cloth and how pretty they are. Put them up and fully appreciate what you've done. Give yourself a fine pat on the back and reward yourself with a cup of tea.

The promise of taking a little time each day in this very aware, awake state has a wonderful balancing effect. You can do this any time no matter what chaos or difficulty may be challenging you. Mindfulness makes you more acutely attuned to yourself. Your feelings and sensations are no longer a mystery and somehow you are more easily able to cope with the wide array of tasks that await you. You are likely to notice a sense of fullness that is very special and most renewing. You are really living your life, not sacrificing even one precious moment for a future that may or may not ever be.

Try not to fear spontaneity. Having our

lives well scheduled and planned is necessary for accomplishing tasks for sure, but don't deny the natural unfolding of yourself in pursuit of this ideal. Realize that life has constant changes in store. Don't be fooled into believing that your schedule can overcome what may jump into its path, nor get bent out of shape when it does. This is just your life in progress, so be it.

According to Hanh,
Everyday we are engaged in a miracle we don't even recognize—a blue sky, a white cloud, green leaves, the curious eyes of our child, our own two eyes—all is a miracle. Work is only a part of life. But work is life only when done in mindfulness. Otherwise, one becomes like the person who lives as though dead. Only by practicing mindfulness will we not lose ourselves but acquire a bright joy and peace, only by practicing mindfulness will we be able to look at everyone with the open eyes and mind of love.[2]

As you can see from this short example, anything you do can be turned into a mindfulness meditation—cleaning the kitchen, taking out the garbage, looking at a sunset, walking on the beach, kissing your child goodnight, eating, driving, taking a shower, ironing, sitting in a dentist chair—*anything.* This serves as a reminder that no detail of your life should be missed. All you have to do is focus on what is happening in the moment and be present for whatever is. So anytime you want, you have the option to close your eyes for a few moments, breathe, and then resume whatever you are doing with mindful awareness of every detail. You may be surprised, as I was, how wonderful and centered you will feel.

Simply put, mindfulness is knowing what you are doing when you are doing it. As we are going through the motions of our lives, our minds are anywhere but on what we are doing. This applies, not only to mundane, boring tasks, but even when we're doing something we enjoy. Unlike children who are focused on the sand in their sandboxes, the water in their baths, and their toys and games, adults are anywhere but right here and now most of the time.

Human beings have a difficult time keeping their minds focused in present time when the past and future are so compelling. When we ruminate about the past and worry about the future, we are missing out on our lives in process. As I watched my 11-year old daughter kissing a dolphin's nose at Discovery Cove, I witnessed a moment in which, for her, there was nothing but the experience of that moment, making it something that neither one of us will ever forget.

Thinking back to your childhood, aren't there memories that are so rich and vibrant that they make up the best parts of the fabric of your being? Images of catching butterflies with Uncle Herman and playing the game, "Two little kids on a deserted island" with my brother, Skip, come to mind. I have such vivid recollections of dressing up in crisply ironed dresses, patent leather shoes and flower adorned hats for church on Easter morning. The scent of lilies and hyacinths brings me back there, to this day. How about standing over an air grate on a hot summer's day in the city and experiencing the warm air rushing up your legs and poofing your dress, or the numbing chill of being the first one into the icy water on a North Atlantic beach. These memories are as clear to me as actually being there, possible only because of the extent of mindfulness given to the details of those moments. This is how children experience life. They laugh, have more fun, and feel more intensely because they are so present. The details of adult life are often so mind numbing that our ability to experience things in this way is exceedingly rare.

John Lennon said, "Life is what happens to you while you are busy making other plans."[3] Have you ever noticed that when you are in the midst of doing something that you have planned and worked for, your mind is already busy thinking about what comes next? The point is the present moment is the only time that we can be 100 percent certain that we will have. So being here now makes your experience and life more vivid and real. So, what is mindfulness? It is nothing more than paying attention to what is going on right now.

Think of all we're missing out on as we race through our lives. Sometime, on a warm spring afternoon, wander out into your yard or a park, using all of your senses, pay close attention to everything around you. Notice the butterfly as it flies around a flowery shrub; notice the colors, the amazing artistic detail of its wings, the lightness with which it flutters, the aroma, and the intricate design and colors of the flowers. Our world is full of such beautiful things, ours for the sensing, yet we rarely take the time to experience them. When did you last really look at a vase full of tulips or the fluffy white clouds turning pink in a blue sky with the setting sun? It's all there, free of charge, yours for the taking. All it requires is awareness, consciousness, and mindfulness. Children do it spontaneously; we need to work at it. Mindfulness meditation is a practice that helps us do just that.

Mindfulness is a reminder to live our lives consciously in each moment instead of reacting automatically. Nadine Stair, at age 85, wrote, "Oh I've had my moments, and if I had it to do over again, I'd have more of them. In fact, I'd have nothing else, just moments, one after another, instead of living so many years ahead of each day."[4]

Even our personal relationships suffer from a lack of mindful attitude. We're all guilty of "yes dear-ing" our spouses and putting off our children with an "ah-huh", or "not right now." We embrace them without really being there. We listen to them but we don't register what has been said. We look at them but we don't see who they are or how they feel. The demands of our busy lives leave only remnants of ourselves to share with those we love, yet, sadly, this is our reality.

Certainly, there are moments when we are fully present, such as a mother's attentiveness to her newborn baby, or when the tears of a child touch her heart, making these the times that we remember. But how much more do we forget? When my daughter, Sarah, was little, I would give her a back massage as her bedtime ritual. She never let me get away with anything, however, as when she sensed that my mind was other than with her, she would complain that I just wasn't doing it right. On those evenings when I was completely present with her, we both benefited.

My brother-in-law, Dave, is my mindfulness guru. When he is with our children, he is *really* with them. Some of their most treasured childhood memories will be of pretending to be human fountains with their Uncle Dave in the pool, his reading to them during long car rides, or helping them make creative claymation movies on the computer, and making up and singing silly songs about our dogs. In truth your presence is the greatest gift that you have to give another person, and Dave has given my children the best gifts of their childhood.

In a recent lecture, one of the participants, saddened by the impending loss of her best friend to ovarian cancer, communicated the sense of helplessness that we have all felt when someone close to us is dying. The need to do something is so strong, yet what can a person do in a situation which seems so hopeless?

This is where your mindful presence is the best gift you could possibly give. Just being there, available to assist with the moment-to-moment desires and discomforts is more than enough. It could be as simple as fluffing a pillow, applying skin cream to itchy dry skin, giving a sip of ginger ale, running to the store when your friend craves the taste of a spicy gumdrop, holding a hand, or applying a cool cloth to a brow; such simple things are wonderful gifts.

The most difficult but crucial part of caring for someone who is ill or near death is accepting what is, then being there for whatever it brings. Often, our desire to keep a friend hopeful and happy through the process comes across as an inability or unwillingness to be present for her reality, thus, making her feel alone in this time of transition. All we need is to be where she is, not where we want her to be. Just sitting in meditative silence while your friend sleeps provides the spacious backdrop that assures her that she can tell you anything, share her thoughts about life, as well as her fears, and perhaps insights about death. Such spaciousness encourages her to finish unfinished business and contemplate her life and eminent transition, and know that she will not be alone. There is nothing better than unconditional, abiding and present love.

If I had to think of one trait that made Mother Teresa the saint that she is, it would be her total love and mindful attention to everyone that she touched. It is apparent even in pictures that each baby she held, each elderly person she comforted, or whomever she was with at any given moment was the only person in her world, and had her full love, caring and mindful attention.

My best days at work are when I focus only on the patient who is sitting in the exam room with me. Though there may be 10 other patients waiting, no one benefits if my attention is somewhere else. It's times like these that I really love being a doctor. There isn't a person in our lives who wouldn't benefit from increased mindfulness, and what better reason to practice being mindful in your meditation practice?

Factory work, housework, or other repetitive jobs can be more fulfilling if done mindfully. It is amazing how paying attention to every detail of cleaning a kitchen, for example, makes it a richer experience. With three kids, three dogs and a tribe of neighborhood friends over most of the time, it feels as though I do this non-stop. Next time you clean off the table, wash the dishes, take out the trash, put food away, or place flowers on the windowsill, be mindful of the details. You may notice that the work goes more quickly and is actually relaxing, making a mundane chore, a rich experience.

Do you remember June Cleaver, of *Leave it to Beaver* fame, clad in heels, a starched cotton shirtwaist dress, coiffed and with full make-up while vacuuming, dusting and joyously preparing meals for Ward, Wally and the Beav? Those of us who came of age in the sixties and seventies looked upon this homemaker prototype of the fifties with disdain for the commitment these women had to home and hearth. In our view, only women who were educated with successful careers were worthy of our respect, setting us up to be career, home and family superwomen. Although many of us actually have pulled it off, it doesn't come without a price. Instead of being mindful of our homes, family, or careers, we're not fully experiencing it.

Many women, now in the early 21st century, are seeing the amazing value that a good mother has in our society. A mindful return to simplicity is in everyone's best interest. Having said that, I can't imagine giving up being a wife, mother, doctor, writer or lecturer, as I thoroughly enjoy each role. But each of these roles can't help but benefit from paying more mindful attention to them. Each of us has the right to make the choices that are best for ourselves. Society, whatever its views at any given time, shouldn't have the power to choose for us.

At Disney World, (some people go to monasteries in India, others climb Mount Everest, I get enlightened at Disneyworld, go figure), I discovered that another use of mindfulness is its ability to settle fear and anxiety. Being phobic about amusement park rides even as fast as a carnival whip (during which I once prayed for God to take me), I wasn't sure how I would fare on Space Mountain with an 11-year old girl whose very personality is a thrill ride. So, I tried an experiment. I decided I would experience Space, Splash and Thunder Mountains in a meditative frame of mind. I knew I had to put my fears aside both to care for my daughter and for important scientific inquiry. To my amazement, I perceived that the rides slowed down both when I closed my eyes and focused on my breathing and when I opened my eyes and mindfully focused on every twist, turn, jolt and plummet. This was in stark contrast to my non-meditative left brain approach during which I was certain that death or at the very least a myocardial infarction was imminent. After numerous rides, it didn't matter any more. My point, however, is that mindful awareness, even of things that scare you, not only makes the experience more tolerable, but also has the potential of making it a relaxing experience. I have done this even in the dentist's chair where paying attention to what is going on in the present moment is not nearly as bad as contemplating what is coming next. Try it.

There is probably nowhere we are less mindful than when we are eating. Often, especially when we are rushed, stressed or too busy to give our bodies proper nourishment and rest, eating becomes a habit. Cramming bags of chips, M&M's or large scoops of peanut butter into our mouths is not truly enjoyable when you really think about it. Although this way of eating temporarily fills the empty spaces caused by skipping meals, anxiety, stress, or depression, we are not nourished in any meaningful way and the mood behind the gluttonous behavior is not addressed. Furthermore, when we are anxious, depressed or lonely, we are physiologically disconnected from our body's feedback loop which is there to tell us that we are full. Therefore, we eat beyond fullness until we feel sick. Psychological detachment from our bodies allows us to consume excessive sweets, alcohol, and fatty foods that we would naturally limit if we were mindful of how it made our bodies feel. I am as guilty of this unhealthy behavior as anyone else is, so I know what I am talking about.

When one eats mindfully, it is a richer, more enjoyable experience. Smaller amounts of quality food are more satisfying when attention is paid to every detail of the experience. You also tend to stay away from foods that make you uncomfortable, as your body's wisdom makes it clear what is not good for you. So mindful eating is actually a two-part process in which you are paying attention to tastes, smells, colors, and textures of the food you are eating; you are also attending to how each part of your body responds to what you put into it. This makes your food truly nourishing as it is meant to be.

You may be thinking that you don't have enough time to eat in this sensuous way. That may be true, but at least attempt to tune in as often as possible and you will see what a difference it makes. On the days that I work from home, I have a mindful bowl of cereal—raisin bran and soy milk—where I pay attention to each taste, texture, temperature and sensation. It is often the best meal of my day and it only takes me five minutes to eat. With eating, as with life, it is not time but consciousness that we lack. Even a glass of cold water, if mindfully consumed, can allow one to choose to wait for a healthy dinner rather than indulging in a junk food appetizer.

Meditation Practice: Mindful Eating

Go to the kitchen and cut yourself a small piece of fruit. A chunk of fresh pineapple is ideal, but an orange, apple or pear slice, or even a raisin will do. Take a few deep mindful breaths and focus on your fruit. Notice its size, shape and color. Is it juicy? Does it have a scent? Look it over carefully until you have witnessed every detail of its appearance. Next, bring it to your lips. Notice its temperature and the sensations on your lips. Is it acidic? Does it sting a little? Does it make your mouth pucker? Now take a tiny bite and slowly chew. Notice every detail of your experience. Does it taste sweet, sour, plain or spicy? Close your eyes, breathe, and slowly consume the whole piece of fruit. What do you notice about this experience? How different would your experience with food be if you allowed yourself to eat this way all the time?

I like to use fresh pineapple in my lecture series for this exercise. After this class, I suspect that the local supermarkets have a rush on pineapples, so impressed are my students that they have just eaten the best pineapple ever grown. Obviously, there is nothing magical about my pineapple; it's all about consciousness. Mindfulness, without a doubt is the best way to experience eating and every part of your life.

So you see, mindfulness is a completely different way of living in which one recognizes the importance of each and every moment. Understand that it isn't just about taking the time to smell the roses; mindfulness must encompass everything in our lives, the good and the bad. Life *is* a mixture of good and bad, beautiful and ugly. Each moment has the possibility of bringing sadness or joy; mindfulness is a practice of embracing both extremes. We tend judge what is good and what is bad. In meditation, we work at being aware of what is without judgment. We suffer when situations in our lives do not go exactly as we planned. The amount of suffering we have is directly related to how attached we are to certain outcomes. In mindfulness meditation, we practice letting go of those expectations and learn to accept circumstances just as they are.

I adopted my three children from Korea. It is the most amazing experience to go to the airport and have someone hand you the baby, who is going to be your child. Not unlike giving birth, you have no idea whatsoever as to who this little human being is or who he or she will become.

So far, I have written the most about my youngest, Sarah, because in many ways, she is intrinsically the most shocking. From the moment she jumped into my arms at six months of age, bent and squirmed around so as not to miss a thing at the airport, crawled around in the back of the limo we rented for this occasion, it was clear that she knew who she was and I would have little impact. Voted in my neighborhood, very shortly after her arrival, 'most likely to be tattooed and/or pierced at an early age', I knew I faced the challenge of my life. As she stood diapered, wearing swim goggles upside down, a dinosaur hat, toting a bazooka-like squirt gun in one hand, her bathing suit swinging wildly in the other, I realized with relief that I wasn't attached to having a quiet, pink-ruffle dressed little girl whose main joy is life was having dainty little tea parties with Mom. If I was attached to her being a certain way, this little girl would have been a scary proposition and she and I would never have a moment's peace. Fantasies about parenting a little angel were short lived when on her first Halloween, the costume she picked for herself was a bright red, pitchfork-carrying, horn-bearing devil. Even though she is my youngest, Sarah is the one who has taught me my most important lesson about accepting what is. Although parenting requires our best efforts at socialization and teaching values, it also requires open armed, loving acceptance of the person that your child is.

Luckily, I am married to a man who is similarly accepting, not batting an eye when our son went through a phase of wearing a fluffy, light blue tutu. Attachment to having a rough and tumble little guy, sporting football paraphernalia would have led to unnecessary suffering. My own attachment kicked in when he actually did become a football player and I was attached to his not being injured; but that's another story.

According to Buddhist philosophy, attachment is the root cause of all suffering. It is not that bad things sometimes happen that makes us unhappy, it is our attachment to thinking things should be different. Westerners find this way of thinking confusing. I am often asked, does this mean that we should never get attached to anyone or anything? My answer to that is no; this is the most rich part of our human experience. Of course, we will be attached to those we love but we must also accept the suffering that will follow if something happens to them or if they are not exactly the way we want them to be. The amount you suffer is directly related to your level of attachment. That's just the way it is.

Mindfulness meditation helps you to accept all things just as they are. By silently witnessing our lives and letting go of judgments, we practice letting go of the attachments which don't serve us and therefore we suffer less. One must also understand that suffering is a part of the human experience, so even our judgment that suffering

48

itself is a bad thing must be suspended.

Our lives are composed of all extremes. Thus, being mindful includes full awareness and acceptance of good and bad, discomfort and comfort, tension and peace, success and failure. The eastern yin-yang philosophy and symbol teaches that the whole is made up of good and bad, darkness and light. Within the bad, there is some good, and within the good, there is some bad. This is a necessity because without sadness, how could we appreciate happiness; and without darkness, there can be no light.

Accepting things just as they are is the secret of a peaceful life. Feeling pain, facing our problems, disappointments and losses head on is the requisite for healing. In mindfulness meditation, we practice this kind of acceptance, making it easier when the inevitable challenges of our lives are before us.

To do a formal mindfulness meditation, find time and a space where you can sit without disruption for a period of peace, quiet and solitude. Meditation is a practice of sitting in restful alertness rather than snoozing in unconscious sleep, so it is best if you sit straight up without having your head supported. Though sitting in the full lotus position would be helpful in preventing one from falling asleep, sitting cross-legged on the beach, on a carpet or in a straight back chair works just as well. Tibetans prefer to keep their eyes open in meditation. But for beginners like me, having eyes closed helps to remain focused. Next, attend to your breathing. Each time your mind wanders just come back to the breath.

Starting with a few moments of breathing is crucial as it anchors your awareness in your body. Think for a moment about what happens when you feel stressed. Your focus of awareness shifts completely out of your body into your mind, where your thoughts and fears totally take over. To regain control, you must center yourself back into your body by breathing, letting your thoughts drift off and witnessing your situation from the center of silence and calm. This will help quiet your conscious mind and in so doing bring you to a place where you can benefit from the wisdom of your very being. Mindful breathing, by itself, moves you from constant doing to just being.

Leo and Flo are a delightful couple, in their seventies, who were attendees at my first lecture series. After each lecture, we would have long philosophical discussions. Leo showed me an advanced understanding of the topic when he said, "I finally got to that place of just being. It was so wonderful. I never wanted to leave that place. And then my thoughts started to intrude; it got me so mad. And then I realized that I usually think so much it hurts." And that is the point— thinking so much that it hurts. Breathing practice minimizes both the thinking and the hurting.

There are two variations on the theme of formal mindfulness meditation. The first is the traditional Tibetan practice that consists solely of focused breathing. In fact, Buddha himself said that if anyone could maintain a perfect breathing focus for a 24-hour period, he or she would become enlightened immediately. Thinking this was worth a try one day, I sat and breathed. Ten seconds later, a thought wandered in. So I started again. Twenty seconds later, another thought. Then, I thought, I'm hungry; what will I make for dinner? Breathe... focus... thought, thought, thought. Perhaps I will become enlightened tomorrow... So as you can see, breathing practice is so simple but so not easy.

The second variation of formal mindfulness meditation is breathing focus and awareness of everything that is in this present moment. Therefore, one attends to breathing as well as all sounds, sensations, bodily sensations and even the thoughts that are a part of each moment in time. This is very different from our usual way of thinking, as in this practice, the task is to be consciously aware of the content of thoughts but not get carried away by them. When thoughts carry us away, awareness ceases. We are thinking constantly, but generally thoughts are just background noise. How often are we actually aware of what we are thinking?

During mindfulness meditation, you pay close attention to each and every thought. After a few moments, your unconscious thought patterns will likely take over. When this happens, your awareness stops dead in its tracks. When you notice that this is happening, gently acknowledge it and return to your breathing. By doing this you become more conscious of your thoughts rather than becoming lost in them.

Meditation Practice: Formal Mindfulness Meditation

Get into a comfortable position in which you can remain alert. Gradually allow your eyes to close and become aware of your breathing. As your thoughts carry you away, re-focus on your breathing. Do this for approximately five minutes.

For the next five minutes, as you continue to focus on your breathing, become acutely aware of bodily sensations, noises, odors and even the thoughts that are a part of the present. If you notice your thoughts carrying you away from awareness, return to the breathing focus.

Following this mindfulness meditation, listen to the following CD meditation which guides you through the process:

Formal Mindfulness Meditation[5]
CD 1, Track 4
Music licensed through Megatrax Production Music, Inc.

"Monkey mind" is a term coined by the Buddhists describing the tendency of our minds to jump from thought to thought just as monkeys swing from tree to tree. This is where most people give up on meditation practice, thinking that they will never be able to achieve the empty mind state that they assume is requisite for good meditation. The fact is, the need to keep pulling your thoughts back over and over again *is* the point. This gives you a lot of practice in calling your thoughts back, making you more likely to be able to focus and concentrate better in your day-to-day tasks especially when stress is causing mental chaos.

Sogyal Rinpoche wrote, "Mind is like an ocean, just as it is. It is the nature of the ocean to rise and fall in waves; it is the nature of the mind to rise and fall in thoughts. The difference between the novice and experienced meditator is that the skilled no longer gets upset about all the thinking. Despite what is going on, on the surface, with meditation you can be as calm underneath as the ocean at its depth."[6]

Meditation requires a stance of nonjudgmental awareness of everything that is in the present moment. Its best use is to provide a quiet, peaceful place from which you can observe your life and be an impartial witness to whatever comes up. This is in stark contrast to our ego mind which will continuously intrude with thoughts like, "this is boring," "this isn't working," "I'm not good enough," "I should be cleaning the house," or even the opposite extreme, "I am now enlightened." None of these thoughts is either helpful or true. You must trust that your inner being will provide you with everything that your mind, body and spirit need. Insights and changes will happen in their own time.

"Beginner's mind" is a Buddhist term referring to the need to enter each meditation completely free of expectation. Perhaps you had an enlightening session or mystical experience, yesterday, only to be disappointed when today's meditation was just boring. I like to think of meditation practice as a treasure chest whose contents change day by day. On some days, it might even be empty. It is always a surprise but, doubtless, replete with meaning of some sort.

The silent witness posture allows you to view physical pain, emotional discord, troubled relationships, and other adversities in your life from a place of equanimity. You will begin to recognize that there is a silent, accepting being inside who, though living comfortably in your body is, in fact, way more than your body. So, if your present moment includes a headache, just observe and accept it. If you are in a bad mood or feeling sad, accept it. If you have been blessed with a wild child instead of a little princess, accept her. Look deeply at your life and everything in it and simply, silently observe and accept your self and your reality just as it is. Accepting things as they are now will help you to accept even more difficult challenges that will undoubtedly happen at some time in the future.

MINDFULNESS

The meditative practice of letting go of thoughts each time they intrude is one that will help you to let go of the problems and worries which have a tendency to consume you. The ability to let go is crucial. Everything in our lives is impermanent. Youth, health, relationships, wealth and your very life are all impermanent phenomena to which your attachment will ultimately cause suffering. Impermanence, another seemingly nihilistic Buddhist philosophy, is reality, pure and simple, the denial of which only makes the situation more difficult than it already is.

The more time and effort you put into this practice, the more benefit you will derive from it. At the Center for Mindfulness at University of Massachusetts (U-Mass) Medical Center, one commits to a 10-week program consisting of a few hours of meditation and weekly instruction, and a commitment to 45 minutes of daily meditation, six days per week. Participants must rearrange their schedules and change their priorities for the program to have maximal impact. The U-Mass program is detailed in *Full Catastrophe Living* by Jon Kabat Zinn and is well worth reading.

According to Kabat-Zinn, the benefits of regular practice are mental stability and resilience, better concentration and focus. Acceptance of your body and life just as it is allows you to suffer less than running away. The more you practice, the better. Even short periods of mindful awareness and quiet observation of your life by your right brain/subconscious mind can help enormously.

After practicing mindfulness, you will find that you are paying a lot more attention to everything in your life and you will start to recognize the beauty that has always existed all around you.

The Center for Mindfulness at U-Mass Medical Center treats people with a variety of medical and chronic pain syndromes for which traditional medicine has been unsuccessful. In one study, symptoms were compared before and after the 10-week meditation program. At the end of the program, participants reported 36 percent fewer symptoms, 50 percent reduction in pain, 30 percent reduction in negative body image, significant reduction in use of pain medications, and 55 percent reduction in anxiety, depression and somatic complaints.

In a four-year follow up, most of the gains reported were

maintained or improved by a continuance of meditation practice. The study found that 95 percent of pain patients kept up some level of meditation practice; 42 percent are still practicing formally three times per week for at least 15 minutes. As compared to standard medical treatment, patients reported that pain improvement was maintained in 35 percent, whereas those treated with traditional pain medications reported no improvement. Meditation improved body image by 37 percent, mood states by 88 percent and psychological distress by 77 percent, as opposed to traditional medical modalities, whose improvements were 1 percent, 22 percent, and 11 percent, respectively.[7]

So, what is it about paying attention that makes such a difference in our perception of our health, if not our actual health status? How much of your life is spent just going through the motions without any actual contact with your experience? Touching without feeling, looking without really seeing, eating without tasting, listening without hearing is more the rule than the exception. Like being on automatic pilot, we go through our lives unaware of how our bodies are affected by our emotions and stress—no connection being made between these things and the headaches, muscle spasm, stomach upset, and hypertension which are a direct result.

The effect of poor food choices, second hand smoke, environmental pollution, and toxic people go unnoticed while our bodies get beat up and sick. Pain and symptoms are the only way that our inner beings have to get our attention. Yet we carry on never paying attention, or making the connection, therefore never addressing the problems that are most likely responsible for our physical distress.

Stress related illness primarily comes about because we are not paying attention. Ultimately, this causes physiologic dis-regulation and yes, actual physical illness. Mindfulness meditation connects you to your body, resulting in physiologic regulation. You don't even have to solve all your life's problems; often just letting your body know that you are listening is enough to diminish or even alleviate your symptoms.

A good way to start is to pay attention to when you are hungry and when you are full. Take a little break when you are tired, have a drink when you are thirsty and use the bathroom, even if you are busy.

Stiff morning muscles are begging to be exercised and stretched, and being grumpy may simply be a plea for more sleep. Perhaps those headaches you get everyday at work are not actually due to that brain tumor you have been secretly fretting about but are trying to tell you that you must figure out a healthier way of dealing with that annoying person who sits next to you at work. Comments such as, "he is such a pain in the neck" and "I can't stomach this anymore" aren't just expressions; they are an accurate assessment of those things in our lives that actually make us sick.

Awareness of these connections allows you to take definitive action to change the problematic situations in your life or to accept them as they are, but to let go of the reactions to them that are making you sick. Without awareness, your only other recourse is to ask your doctor for a prescription that may, if you are lucky, make it go away with no effort on your part. Mindful awareness of your body and sought after assistance from your doctor is giving it your best shot.

No one disagrees that pain and illness create stress, and that stress creates more pain and illness—a vicious cycle that can stop only with awareness. Pay attention to how you relate to your pain. If you have a headache, is your reaction, "Oh my God, I have this headache again. It will never go away. I won't be able to go to work like this. I can't stand my children's noise. Who will raise them when I die of that aneurysm that I just know is responsible for this headache?" Contrast this to a mindful approach which is to grab a few Advil, (yes, that is OK), then sit, close your eyes, breathe, and ask, "Oh there you are again, headache, what are you trying to tell me today?" Once you get used to approaching your symptoms in this fashion, you will be amazed at the answers that will flash before your mind's eye. Not only that, but there is an excellent chance that just stopping, breathing, resting, and inquiring will help alleviate many headaches even in the absence of answers.

An important function of mindfulness meditation practice is that it gives you the opportunity to listen to your body. "Never let a good symptom go to waste" is advice that I now give to all of my patients. This is surely a different way of looking at things. Since you will have physical and emotional symptoms throughout your life anyway, you might as well learn something about yourself by asking if this symptom has any meaning. Quietly ask the symptom, "What are you here for?" The challenge is to see if we can interpret these messages and use them to make positive changes in our lives. This is a way of facing your problem head on, not only accepting it, but looking deeply into its meaning.

The up side of impermanence is that unpleasant things, like pain, are impermanent too. Understand that no matter what you are going through in this moment, it will be gone the next. When you observe your problems, be they physical, emotional, or spiritual, through the eye of your silent witnessing inner being, you will come to realize that, despite what is happening to your body, the real you is and will always be perfectly fine. Jon Kabat-Zinn refers to this phenomenon as "encountering your intrinsic wholeness."

A good way to work with your body and pain in meditation is to use the body scan. Scanning your body as you breathe helps you center your awareness in your body. It is also a chance for you to express your gratitude for all the parts that work well and provides the opportunity to question your symptoms system by system.

To do this, close your eyes. Focus on your breath. Move your mind through each part of your body, feeling every area and every sensation. Directing your breath to each area increases your awareness. Awareness in and of itself may even provide symptom relief. Breathing can also be used as a kind of purification process in which you use the image of breathing energy and health in and breathing pain and fatigue out to work with your pain.

Body Scan with Symptom Focus
CD 1, Track 5
Music Licensed through Megatrax Production Music, Inc.

A similar process can be used for anything that is causing you pain. Emotional stress caused by relationships, work or just having too much on your plate, can all be helped by viewing them from that place of inner silence. Say, for example, you are feeling depressed. Mindfulness meditation gives you a way to face and accept it just as it is. With your conscious mind quieted, you have the opportunity to inquire deeply into the emotion and learn from it. There is no guarantee that you will come out of your meditative session a brand new happy person, but with each attempt, you will gain more insight into its cause and to possible solutions. If there is nothing you can do to change the situations in your life that are causing you to feel depressed, taking the time to observe it from a center of equanimity will help you to make peace with what cannot be changed. So often we are just in pain; consciousness keeps us from becoming its victim.

Everyone faces illness, sadness and tragedy; such is the human condition. It is easy, however, to make things worse than they need to be. Running away and wanting things to be different than they are is the usual response, thus causing more pain than the original problem ever could. Facing the problem in silence helps one to understand when decisive action can be taken or when total surrender or peaceful acceptance is the best course.

Your meditation practice on emotional pain is a period of silent awareness in which you sit with the emotion, breathe into it, welcome it into your consciousness and don't try to push it away. Focusing on the problem rather than fretting about it allows you to understand its causes, take action when possible, or make peace with it. Understand that *everything* in your life is okay when it is experienced quietly by your inner being – EVERYTHING!

Remember being taught that you should count to 10 before engaging in a tirade? Perhaps stopping for a few mindful breaths would be better as it engages your peaceful, loving right brain that can help to modulate an irate left brain when you are angry. By taking you away from the heat of the moment, breathing allows the introspection that helps you to see your own responsibility in the conflict. Flying off the handle and attacking another without first examining your own thoughts, feelings and behaviors will never lead to a peaceful resolution. Your right brain's input will lead to a discussion which is less hurtful and condemning to yourself and to the other person.

For those of you who are parents and use this as an excuse not to have a meditation practice, Jon Kabat-Zinn considers parenting to be the perfect 20-year mindfulness retreat. In his book, *Everyday Blessings,* Jon compares children to Zen masters. Like the teachers of Zen Buddhism, children make us look at ourselves. They teach us lessons, point out our weaknesses, and are not always gentle about it. They push every button. The fact that we have buttons to push probably says more about us and our own coping abilities than about our children. Children have a way of challenging everything we believe in, especially during those adolescent/teenage years when your ability to remain calm is pushed beyond its limit. Whatever we consider to be reasonable goals or attitudes will be challenged, as this is a time when they are making their own way and their own statements. Their need to reject parental opinion, even if it is in their own best interest, is a necessary and horrifying stage in our children's lives as well as our own; our attachments exposed, we suffer accordingly.

From infancy to adulthood, our children have constantly changing needs of which we must be mindful. If you think you have it all figured out with your first child, think again; each child is a completely different entity, requiring ultimate flexibility in your approach to parenting him/her. Even though we are beyond busy with jobs, homes, and details of keeping everything together, children require that we be fully present and will get our attention one way or another if we are not. Parental responsibilities never stop; problems must be faced head on and dealt with, and there is no hiding. Raising children is wonderful and terrible, happy and sad, fun and really no fun at all, yin and yang; thinking otherwise will cause suffering. The only way to get through this is to make sure that you take care of yourself, recharge your batteries and use your whole brain—right and left—to do the job. Meditation provides a solution.

I return to the concept of choice. Our lives are full of choices. We make some for better, others for worse. We know we can choose to live in this house or that, go to college or not, get married and have children or remain single. But what isn't apparent to most of us is that happiness itself is something which we can choose...or not.

The choice to live a more mindful life and practice mindfulness meditation guarantees a happier life for you and for everyone you touch. We gain equanimity by accepting our lives just as they are and understanding that change, illness, death or impermanence, in whatever form it takes, is an integral part of our lives, posing no actual threat to who we really are.

58

MINDFULNESS

Mindfulness helps us to understand that there is no point in trying to control the uncontrollable. Sitting with things just as they are is the only true road to peace. You can choose to look at a storm with its dramatic lightning flashes and thunder either as a magnificent, powerful, beautiful force of nature, or you can run and hide under your bed fearing that the next flash will cause your home and family to go up in flames; the choice is yours. Losing your job can be viewed as a tragedy or an opportunity to pursue the vocation of your dreams; it's all a matter of interpretation. If I had spent valuable time ringing my hands and bemoaning my fate over my infertility, I would have missed the opportunity to adopt three incredible children. I would have missed the chance to experience the love that only parenting can provide. I would have missed the lessons that they teach me everyday, and missed out on having children who couldn't be more mine even if I had given birth to them. Making positive choices is difficult as long as one stays trapped in trying to change that which simply cannot be changed. Once peace is made with what is true, choices leading to happiness naturally follow.

A mindful approach to life presumes the understanding that everything that we need for happiness is right here in this present moment. Like a person sitting next to a beautiful clear fresh waterfall and dying of thirst because he doesn't have anything resembling a Poland Springs bottle, we often miss the fact that what we need most is no further away than a few mindful breaths. We are fooled into believing that happiness will be ours when we can buy that house, boat or new car, or if we could only take that Caribbean vacation. Perhaps a diamond ring or an in-ground pool will finally bring the contentment that we seek. Although these things are wonderful, the pleasure they provide is often short lived and devoid of any real meaning. True happiness is a lot closer and doesn't cost anything. What is required is that we look inside ourselves. Guillaume Apollinaire wrote, "Now and then it's good to pause in our pursuit of happiness and just be happy."

When one is truly mindful, he understands that happiness is an inside job; no one can do it for you. There is no place better than right here; there is no better time than right now. When you grasp the concept of mindfulness, you realize that what really counts can be found by sitting, breathing, and just being. When all is said and done, it is self-knowledge and living a life that is congruent with who you really are which brings the happiness that is your birthright. Happiness has very little to do with what we have but everything to do with who we are and the choices we make. Transformation of painful human existence begins and ends with connecting in silence to our own true nature where our lives and our selves are perfect just as they are.

CHAPTER SEVEN

Imagery

Preconceived notions of what imagery is all about can interfere with trying this very useful practice. People often come into this practice thinking this is something that one must be skilled at or creative to use. I am often told, "I can't do imagery, I can't see things." If your expectation is one of visualizing clear vibrant psychedelic colored images, then you are probably correct. Short of taking mind-altering substances, this will most likely not happen. Images may be as clear as an impressionistic painting for some, and for others they will just be a vague visual impression.

As with any type of meditation, there is no magic and no particular skill involved. Imagery is what you picture, sense or feel when you close your eyes and think. It is nothing more than your own inner representation of thoughts, emotions, or your outer experiences. Though we usually think of images as visual phenomena, they are actually multi-sensory and can be heard, tasted, smelled or felt. As with visual images, these may not be sensed to the degree that actually smelling or hearing something in our environment would be, but one has the impression of engaging all five senses.

All of your thoughts are images. Words themselves are only verbal representations of what in fact are images of the ideas we have in our minds. The following is an exercise that will give you a clearer idea of how you experience images.

Imagery practice: Mini Visualizations
CD 1, Track 6

Were you able to sense the various images as they were presented to you? Did you notice how flexible your mind is in its ability to switch from image to image? This is exactly how your images will appear to you in imagery meditation. The fact is you do imagery all the time. Thoughts, plans and worry are all images that we do everyday with no particular thought or skill required. I would be willing to bet that there isn't a person reading this book who doesn't know how to worry. If you can worry, you are an absolute pro at imagery!

Worry is the most common form of imagery because it goes on all the time. It requires no particular effort or consciousness on our part that it is even happening. Unfortunately, even though we may not be aware of it, our health is adversely affected by nothing more than the insidious, troubling worry images that provide the foundation for many of our decisions and actions throughout the day. Recalling the fight flight response, worry, by itself, is sufficient to initiate the entire bio-physiologic stress cascade with all its physical ramifications. Thankfully, most of our worst worries never actually materialize. But because of the ease with which the stress response is activated, our bodies get beaten up as if each worry image is an actual event.

At one time or another, we all go through periods of habitual worry, some more than others. Jumping from one obsessive concern to the next, one enters a never-ending process leading to exhaustion, burn out, physical symptoms, depression, and stress. The only threat in these situations is our thoughts, which are nothing more than images which have sadly taken on lives of their own, leaving us feeling terribly out of control.

In other words, what you habitually think (or your ongoing imagery) has significant effects on your body. Remember, worried images lead to stress. This produces a physiologic stress response and initiates the production of unhealthy neuropeptides. But the good news is that images consisting of joy and relaxation produce the physiologic relaxation response and healthy neuropeptides with all the associated positive health benefits.

Images are so powerful that the PET scan of a person who is actually looking at an object is the same as the scan of someone who is just imagining it. Steven Kosslyn of Harvard Medical School has shown that MRI and SPECT scans show that imagining a visual image lights up the occipital cortex, an auditory image lights up the temporal lobe, and imaging yourself moving activates the prefrontal cortex. These areas of the brain are activated in the same way as they would be if the person were actually seeing an image, hearing a sound or moving.[1]

"Going to your happy place," a phrase generally used in jest, is actually an important use of imagery. Picturing yourself at the beach, for example, where you feel happy and relaxed has the same effect on your brain as actually being there. This causes positive changes in your brain's biophysiology and leads to positive changes in the physiology of your body. So, it turns out that "going to your happy place" is actually a great idea.

Hans Eysenk did a study in England looking at the psychological profiles of 13,000 people. Group 1 was the "Hopeless Group," representing people who were depressed; feeling as though could never have what they wanted. Group 2 was the "Angry Group." This group tended to blame others for their unhappiness. Group 3 was made up of people who felt self-actualized, believing that happiness comes from one's own actions and attitudes and is essentially an inside job. In other words, group 1 had constant images of hopelessness, Group 2's images were angry; and Group 3 had images of contentment and being in charge of their own destinies. Of the people who ultimately died of cancer, 75 percent were from the depressed group, 15 percent from the angry group, and less than 1 percent from Group 3. Of the patients who died of heart disease, the opposite was true. 15 percent were from Group 1, 75 percent from Group 2, and again less than 1 percent from Group 3.[2] What this shows is that people who carry around depressed, hopeless images will be at more risk for cancer. Those whose images are angry will have a greater likelihood of having heart trouble, and those whose ongoing imagery involves taking responsibility for their own happiness are far and away more likely to die during old age. These scenarios don't always apply, but there is a definite trend.

Hopefully, you are beginning to see how powerful your thoughts/images are. The good news is that you can consciously change your images to ones that will help you to be healthier and happier. In the *Dhammapada*, the Buddha says, "Mind is the forerunner of all things. As we think and act so our world becomes." You can see this is more than just a supposition or a philosophy; scientific research is proving it right down to a cellular level.

How can one change images or thoughts when going through difficult times? On some level, aren't we just passive victims to whatever may befall us? If that is true, how does one explain Anne

Frank's attitude during the holocaust? In Diary of a Young Girl, she wrote,

> *I keep my ideals because in spite of everything, I still feel that people are really good at heart. I simply cannot build up my hopes on a foundation of confusion, misery and death. I can feel the sufferings of millions and yet if I look up into the heavens, I think that it will come right that this cruelty too will sometime end and that peace and tranquility will return to the earth.* 3

Now that's imagery! Clearly, this young woman had no objective evidence that humans were basically good; quite the contrary. However, the fact that she had these positive images not only helped her to survive under adverse circumstances, but to live a life which was fulfilled to the extent that generations of people would have the chance to benefit from her amazing spirit through her writing.

Take a moment to inventory your own internal images. Are you an optimistic person who accepts life as it comes and understands that all things happen as they are supposed to? Or, do you feel that life throws you one curve ball after another and nothing ever goes your way? Do you see life as interesting, replete with amazing possibilities for self-actualization, or as something which has to be survived day after dismal day? Are you able to face your life and those in it with a warm smile, or is a hostile sneer your more likely approach? How you answer these questions determines what your reality will be. But what you may not realize is the importance that choice plays in these attitudes.

Jack Kornfield, an American Buddhist teacher and practitioner, tells the story about a wise old sage who was walking along the road one day. After a while, a man stopped his vehicle, told the old man that he was moving into town, and wondered what the people were like there. The old man asked, "What were they like where you came from?" The man answered, "They were, warm and friendly; I had so many wonderful friends there." The old sage said, "You will find exactly the same thing here." As the sage walked further, another driver stopped and asked the same question. Again, the old man asked,

"How were the people where you came from?" The driver answered, "They were mean, selfish, and unfriendly." Upon hearing this, the sage replied, "You will find them to be the same here"; demonstrating the point that your attitude determines how you will view your reality. **You do not see the world as it is; you see the world as you are.**

Doesn't it make sense then to practice forms of meditation that have the possibility of changing your internal images from sad to happy, pessimistic to optimistic, angry to forgiving, hateful to loving, ugly to beautiful, devastating to profound?

One way that imagery meditation can help is to recognize that worries, obsessions and negative thought patterns are nothing more than images. With conscious effort, it is possible to replace worry images with peaceful images. And amazingly enough, changing worry images to peaceful images can change you biophysiologically from stressed to relaxed. **YOU ALWAYS HAVE A CHOICE.**

Just like practicing the relaxation response, sending your subconscious mind joyful, loving, peaceful and relaxing images initiates multiple sequences of physiologic events that enhance each and every system of your body.

What is so special about images? Why can't a person just intellectually change his attitude? One can change one's attitude, certainly something to be encouraged. The problem is that only the central nervous system (responsible for voluntary movement or action) responds to ordinary thoughts. In order to affect the autonomic nervous system, (responsible for involuntary functions such as heartbeat and blood pressure), one must use images. Autonomic bodily functions will not respond to conscious commands but do seem to be affected by the images sent to them.

How do we know that this is true? Don't you blush when you have an embarrassing thought? All it takes is the image of something embarrassing to cause the blood vessels in the face to dilate, causing a red blush. You can't consciously command your face to blush; it doesn't work that way. This next example further illustrates this point.

Meditation Practice: Effect of Imagery on the Autonomic Nervous System

Take a few deep breaths. Do a quick survey of your body. Notice what your feet, ankles and legs feel like. Feel the weight sitting on your buttocks. Sense your abdomen, chest, and back. Notice your arms, and any sensations you are having there. Now become aware of your neck and head. As you continue to breathe, do the sensations in any of these areas change?

Now that you are feeling relaxed, visualize going to your refrigerator, opening the door, peeking into the fruit drawer and seeing a lemon. Notice the bright yellow color. Now put your hand in and gently lift the lemon out of the drawer. Feel its texture, feel the coolness. Carry the lemon over to a cutting board and cut it into quarters. Can you smell the lemon oil scent? Notice the cool juice on your fingers. As you are doing this, do you notice anything happening to your body? What do you notice? Gently pick up one of the lemon quarters, bring it to your nose and smell it? Now place your lips on the pulp of the lemon and bite. What do you notice? What are the sensations in your body? Is this a pleasant sensation? What is happening to the saliva in your mouth as you imagine this?

Notice how just having the image of the lemon sets off the totally autonomic function of salivating in your body. This is how imagery works.

Joan Borysenko suggests using brief joyful thoughts

throughout the day. Just like spending a little time each day visualizing those things for which you are grateful, taking a few moments to focus on joyful things can affect your mood, attitude and physiology in a positive way. Take a few moments to try the following example.

Meditation Practice: Brief Joyful Thought Imagery Meditation

Take a few relaxing breaths and make yourself comfortable. After a brief body scan, recall something that made you happy— perhaps your baby's first smile, the kindness of a friend or an act of your own kindness. Enter this image with all your senses. What do you see? How do you feel? Can you hear or taste anything different? Are there any special fragrances? Pay attention to how this memory feels in your body. Close your eyes and spend a few moments noticing how your body responds to this image of pure joy.

Physiologically, positive imagery meditation elicits the relaxation response, thus counteracting the effects of the fight-flight response. The formation of euphoric neuropeptides and the activation of neuropeptide receptor sites results. This starts or stops the protein synthesis affecting every system of your body. So every joyful image you have will literally impact every cell of your body.

Imagery has been shown to have many useful purposes. For more information, I recommend *Guided Imagery for Self-Healing* by Martin Rossman, M.D., and research done by Norman Shealy, M.D. Although it has only gotten press in the last few decades, Olympic and professional sports athletes have been using imagery to improve their performance for some time. Dr. Shealy presented a study done in 1970 with weight lifters. In this study, Group 1 lifted a little more weight each day, Group 2 imagined lifting more weight each day, and Group 3 did both. Not surprisingly, Group 3 did the best. But what may surprise you is there was essentially no difference between the abilities of Groups 1 and 2.[4]

In another study, Dr. Shealy worked with a basketball team. Half the players were given imagery meditation exercises where they visualized making baskets every time; the other half did not meditate. The study revealed that the half who used imagery did 80 percent better at free throws than those who didn't.[5] Dr. Shealy also worked with a football team who hadn't had a winning season for many years. He led six 30-minute imagery sessions in which the team pictured their successes in scoring and defense. This team became regional champions that year and continued having successful seasons as the coach kept them meditating year after year.[6]

A recent study done at the Cleveland Clinic tested subjects for strength in the fifth finger and the biceps muscle. Group 1 worked with weight exercises for both areas, and Group 2 did imagery meditation 20 minutes per day for the same length of time. At the end of six weeks, the two groups improved their strength equally.[7]

The U.S. Army did a study in which soldiers were put into a subzero environment. The first group wore thin leather gloves alone. The second group wore the same gloves but was taught meditation focused on keeping their hands warm. The third group was given arctic gloves. Researchers found that Groups 2 and 3 maintained their hand warmth equally.[8] This study describes a self-treatment known as autogenic training, an important feature of biofeedback therapy, in which a person is trained to use his/her mind to make specific changes in the body.

As impressive as these studies are, I wouldn't suggest that simply visualizing running in the Boston Marathon 20 minutes a day for one year would in any way prepare me to jump right into the race without the appropriate physical training. But these studies all show how powerful our minds are, and how our conscious use of them can improve anything that we are doing.

Aside from its influence on your autonomic nervous system, imagery is also the best way to communicate with your subconscious mind. Images are the language of the right brain. Sigmund Freud helped us to understand how important one's subconscious thought processes are in relation to how we feel and what we believe. Along with Carl Jung, Freud recognized that a person's images represent his internal reality. Dr. Assagioli, a contemporary of Freud and Jung, went on further to explain that by tapping into our unconscious (right brain) by means of images, we are able to access our creativity, feelings, compassion, and our source of inspiration.

At this point, a deeper understanding of the differences between the left and right brain may be helpful. The left brain (conscious mind) responds to and understands words. It takes care of our day to day tasks and is responsible for logical, analytical and objective thinking. It is rational and functions well in the material world. The left brain tends to look at things in parts rather than at the whole picture.

The right brain (subconscious mind) is more random and intuitive, highly intelligent, and connected to the emotional realms. More holistic, the right brain tends to see the forest while the left is busy analyzing the trees.

In order to function as a human here on earth, one must have a highly functional left brain. However, to function maximally, the right brain must be accessed for its psychological, emotional and spiritual wisdom.

There are many ways to make the right brain more accessible. I have already written at length about how meditation does this. Hypnosis, often shrouded in a cloud of mystery and magic, is actually similar to meditation. A hypnotherapist performs a hypnotic induction (which is no more than deep relaxation) in which your conscious mind is put to rest. He/she then makes suggestions to your subconscious or right brain. When you are brought out of your hypnotic state, you will have engaged your right brain to assist you in whatever problem you are working on. Imagery meditation is very much like hypnosis, except that you make suggestions to your own subconscious mind by the use of images.

The following meditation exercise demonstrates how the use of images can deepen your relaxation and meditative state. Once relaxed, images are used to actively engage your right brain and quiet the ever busy left brain. With each image, you become more deeply relaxed and more aware of your own inner being and wisdom.

Imagery to Deepen Relaxation[9]
CD #1, Track #7
Music licensed by Megatrax Production Music, Inc.

The ability to communicate with your right brain is particularly important for helping yourself to heal, physically or emotionally. When you think about it, healing is an unconscious process. Say you have a cut on your hand. It will heal without any conscious effort on your part; it just happens. So it makes sense that this process will be better understood by the unconscious part or right brain. To assist in your own healing, it is helpful to send healing images to and to learn how to receive healing information from your right brain, allowing it to contribute its wisdom to the process.

The right brain is the center of emotion. Our ability to experience and express emotions plays a huge role in our health status. A few hundred years ago, Dr. Rudolf Virchow said, "Much illness is unhappiness sailing under a physiologic flag."

A person's inner conflict, problems and concerns, which for one reason or another cannot be expressed, are likely to be expressed in physical symptoms. Say one is staying in a difficult marriage for the sake of children. In order to keep a modicum of peace, emotions are often pushed undercover. Needing to find expression somewhere, our bodies develop physical symptoms as a way of getting us to pay attention to the unhappiness or imbalance in our lives. Failure to attend to the physical symptoms results in more symptoms, sometimes in the dire consequence of serious illness. Dr. Bernie Siegel says, "Be honest with your feelings, your body will respond. Heal your life and there will be physical consequences." Being mindful of your body is the first step in healing. Using imagery to engage your right brain's wisdom in the process gives you the best shot at complete healing.

Emotions also play a role in how we experience our symptoms. In the emergency room, just by observing the patients' emotions, it is very clear to me who will get better quickly and who will have symptoms that will linger and even cause permanent disability. If someone is panicking about what having "a bad back" will mean for his life, he won't likely do very well. If I hear, "Oh my God, how shall I support my family? What if it is a disc? I knew someone who had a disc problem and he never worked again. My mother lived a life of agony because of her bad back," I know that a poor prognosis is likely. As compared to someone who comes in and says, "Yep, I sprained my back again; should be better in a few days. When can I get back to work?" This person will likely get back to normal quickly. Panic and fear cause muscles that are already sore and in spasm to tense even more, increasing the pain. Panic also tends to cause people to hyperventilate, which in and of itself increases muscle spasm.

Take a moment to try this experiment. Close your eyes and start to breathe quickly, then notice what happens to the muscles in your back and neck. Even when pain free, you will observe how the act of hyperventilating causes muscles to tense. One's natural tendency to hyperventilate during actual pain greatly magnifies pain perception. One of the simplest things a person can do to diminish the sensation of pain is to close his eyes, consciously slow down and focus on the breath. Quiet, gentle, slow breathing acts as a natural muscle relaxant. The people who are in pain who do this with my instruction are more likely to leave the ER without any need for pain medication, plus they feel a sense of control over their own bodies.

As always, begin your imagery meditation by arranging a period of silence and solitude. Focus on the breath and perform a body scan. This will get you into your body and away from the usual barrage of thoughts. Focusing on a deepening image, as demonstrated in the last recorded exercise, helps to engage your right brain. You can then use imagery as a way of opening a two-way communication between your conscious mind (left brain) and your subconscious (right brain).

Active imagery is the method of sending messages from your conscious mind to your subconscious mind. You do this by consciously visualizing an image that represents your desired goal, such as picturing yourself at your favorite beach. Or, send the image of your white blood cells as little Pacmen chomping on virus particles with the goal of assisting with recovery from an infection, like a cold. The best images for healing are individual and must make sense to the person who is using them. Research has also shown that the images will be more beneficial if they represent a process which is basically anatomically correct.

71

The most important component of active imagery is that you continually use it. Norman Shealy gives an example of a patient who had an enlarged prostate gland who was told by another physician that a prostatectomy was the only solution. Dr. Shealy gave him the image of his prostate being a big balloon which he was to mentally watch deflate for about twenty minutes each day. Amazingly, in just two weeks, the man's prostate gland had shrunk to normal size and he never required surgery.[10]

Dr. O. Carl Simonton has done many studies demonstrating increased longevity in cancer patients who have used the image of cancer cells being gobbled up by colorful little Pacmen, which is just what our white blood cells should be doing. Active images can be anything you want them to be such as imaging painful muscles as knots untying themselves, or a cool mountain stream bathing a hot acidic ulcer. Many people with cancer have been taught to imagine that their chemotherapy medicines are Star Wars characters blasting away at cancer cells.

I would never recommend that a person neglect traditional medical treatment and only use his imagination to heal. But it seems to me that the concomitant use of imagery gives the patient more of an active role in his/her treatment. By employing every means available, especially the power of the person's own mind, one will obtain the best possible result.

Children are particularly good at imagery healing. Again Dr. Shealy writes of a study he did with children in a burn unit. Half the group was told to imagine little hands reaching up from a burn and holding little hands reaching down from the skin graft; the other half were given no imagery. At the end of six weeks, the children who used imagery had a better chance at a successful graft.[11] According to Shealy, "There is virtually no illness which cannot be reversed or significantly helped by positive attitude, imagery and relaxation."[12]

Images can be imaginary or real and are helpful either way. Joan Borysenko writes about how terminally ill people who have the image of living until meeting a future goal, such as a grandchild's wedding or graduation, will generally live longer than those who have no such goal. She further states that everyone's healing ability would be enhanced by joyful images.

IMAGERY

Bernie Siegel cautions, however, that joy is in the eye of the beholder; what may be a happy image for one person may not work for another. Dr. Siegel tells the story of an elderly, religious patient of his who had been ill for a long time and was ready to meet his maker. One day, the family gathered to say their good-byes, as it was clear that the man was finally coming to the end of his life. According to Siegel, "At that moment, the patient became so overjoyed, he recovered." In this case, just the thought that he would finally finish with his suffering and be with God was enough joyful imagery to make his body temporarily heal. This scenario took place not once, but three times. So never make assumptions about what causes another's happiness.

Why doesn't imagery healing get the attention it deserves from the traditional medical establishment? In defense of my colleagues, they are products of our own materialistic western culture, which is predominantly left-brain and concrete in thought and beliefs. So philosophically, many believe that if you can't see it, can't x-ray it, or can't take it out, it doesn't exist. In contrast, eastern culture is predominantly right-brain and abstract, and is more likely to believe in things that can't be seen, touched or measured (like the movement of chi in acupuncture or qigong for example), and that healing all parts of the person is important. This includes the non-material, even if not amenable to materialistic scientific scrutiny.

Scientific proof is the very heart of western medicine. And though critical for curing the physical body, doesn't necessarily address the emotions, psyche, and soul, which are central to our humanness. This provides a partial explanation of why many people, including my friend Lynn, feel diminished by their medical treatment.

Many people are angry at their doctors for not being more open to holistic, mind-body healing. But I have a theory. First of all, one must understand that the rigors of medical training and practice are such that only the most extremely talented left-brain people make it through. Asking your doctor to have an equally developed right brain or consciousness is like demanding that your favorite professional athlete also be a concert pianist or an acclaimed poet. Although the two aren't necessarily mutually exclusive, they aren't likely to be developed to the same degree in one person. The fact is you really do want someone with a remarkable left brain to be doing your cardiac or brain surgery. You can get the other stuff elsewhere or even better, learn how to take care of your non-physical needs yourself. So be grateful to your doctors for the skills that only they can provide.

Receptive imagery, the reverse of active imagery, provides a way for your subconscious to communicate with your conscious mind. All you need to do is ask your subconscious mind a question and then pay attention to the images that you get in return while in a meditative state. These images may come in the form of thoughts, feelings, sensory images or even in dreams. What is interesting about this process is that, even if you don't get any images during the meditation session in which the question was asked, pay attention over the next several weeks. The answers may come in the form of something you hear on the radio, read in a book, or overhear in a conversation. The important thing is to ask the questions. Trust me, answers will come, one way or another when questions are sincerely asked.

For insight into symptoms or illness, ask your subconscious what this situation is trying to tell you and then receive whatever images it sends back. As mentioned in the chapter on mindfulness, symptoms are not necessarily the enemy. They may be a natural warning; your body's attempt to communicate with you about imbalance in your life. Looking at symptoms as potential blessings in disguise helps you to abandon thoughts like, "Why does this have to happen to me?" and embrace an attitude of, "Since I am going to have this symptom anyway, I might as well learn something from it." Given the impact of one's emotional response to his suffering, which attitude do you think would get a person better faster? With the second, more positive attitude, recovery is not only faster, but what you learn from your illness will impact your well-being for the rest of your life. Discovering the actual cause of the symptom gives you the opportunity to change what needs to be changed in your life or make peace with what cannot. Having served its purpose, the symptom may well go away. So remember, **never let a good symptom go to waste!**

As you work with imagery, be forewarned that you may get images that surprise you. It is very important to use these images as a starting point for your thought process and take the time to consider what they actually mean. Let me give you an example. For many years, I had daily migraine headaches and constant neck pain. I took these symptoms into meditation and asked my subconscious mind, why were these symptoms here and what were they trying to tell me? In an instant, my husband's image flashed before my mind's eye. This came as quite a shock, as everyone who knows him would agree there is no one who is less of a pain in the neck than he is. So my options were to toss him out of my life or contemplate what this image was trying to tell me. Many meditation sessions and journal entries later, the meaning became crystal clear.

In most relationships there are compromises made to keep the peace. Sometimes these compromises are necessary other times they are not. There is a chameleon-like quality to my personality (quite common in most women) that assumes that to please another, I have to become more like him, my own self not being good enough. In order to be more in sync with a sweet, but decidedly logical, left-brained husband, I hid the person I really am. I felt this same transformation was necessary to fit into the western medicine culture in which I found myself. What resulted was a person who barely recognized herself and a body, racked with pain, trying to get the message across that the person that I really am, was literally being crushed. With trepidation, I shared this with my husband, who, contrary to my greatest fear, was delighted. He recognized that the woman he married had changed, and though he understood why, it made him sad. My attempt to be more like him rather than the person he married was exactly what he didn't want. And in truth, my right-brain intuition and emotional accessibility are the real gifts that I bring to my medical practice; it doesn't need to be under cover.

So you see, doing this inner work was time well spent. Now headaches and neck pain are a thing of the past and my relationship with my husband is better than ever. I'm much happier being a doctor, no longer doubting that my real self brings something unique to my patients' healing process. Teaching and writing about what I have always known to be true in my heart, despite disapproval of some traditional medical colleagues, makes my "coming out party" complete. There is nothing better for a person's well-being than unabashedly being him or herself.

The number of internal conflicts with the potential to produce symptoms in people is limitless, and relationships are the most likely

75

source. We have all suppressed anger and frustration to keep peace. Although this may keep a relationship together, it comes at huge personal expense. The fear of being alone, financially unstable, or of having to admit that we made a mistake can keep us in situations which are devastating to our minds, spirits, emotions and bodies. Being "broken hearted" is not just an expression; it may become the physical reality of a relationship which is drowning in anger. Toxic relationships unfortunately do exist.

Symptoms can also appear as physical expressions of repressed trauma or abuse as in people with post traumatic stress syndrome or as a physical manifestation of a poor self-image. It is not unusual for a person to develop symptoms as a way of avoiding overwhelming responsibilities, getting attention or as the only way he or she can justify taking time out to get needed rest. Occasionally, people who feel guilty or responsible for something bad happening can develop symptoms as an unconscious need for self-punishment.

Physical symptoms are likely to manifest in any situation in which a person has compromised himself, such as staying in a job he hates instead of risking financial security by doing what he loves. The happiest and healthiest people are those who take the time required to get to know their true selves and live congruently with who they are.

The reasons for physical symptoms are as many as the people who have them. The only hope that one has of true inner and outer wellness is the willingness to take the time to do the work required. Being very individual, this is something that must be done for and by oneself. Without the work, you have no insight, no control, no clue, and you just have symptoms. Working with what you learn from the images sent from your right brain is one of the best possible ways that you can contribute to your own health and well-being.

Simply giving your subconscious a voice is often enough to make the symptoms go away or at the very least, will help you to examine your life and point you in a healthier direction. Any time you give your subconscious a voice, you will experience peace and equanimity not otherwise possible and you will continuously learn more about what your life is all about. Imagery or meditation does not necessarily promise you a physical cure, nor should you leave your doctor out of this loop. But there is no question that, even in the absence of a cure, using imagery can decrease the symptoms of an illness and the side effects of medications, and empower you to be an active participant in your own treatment.

Lynn had significant symptom relief when she could get herself into a deep relaxed state. She was very skilled at imagery and used it frequently to get through difficult periods. Toward the end of her life, she was tortured by nightmares. One day we tried an experiment in which I helped her get into a deep relaxation, then made the suggestion to her subconscious that each time a nightmare would start, her right brain would immediately transport her to her favorite place—a church in Tuscany which she described to me in detail. This was four weeks before she passed away, during which time she didn't mention any more nightmares.

Even though Lynn was never cured of her cancer, her remarkable skill at introspection helped her to learn a lot about her life and what was important. She would often say that a lot of good things came out of this tragedy. This would have been impossible without the ability to look deeply into herself and find meaning.

Although being right-brain dominant may give one a head start, so to speak, devastating sadness or tragedy has a way of breaking one's heart wide open, bringing him right to the core of his being. No one asks for bad fortune. But if it should arrive, take time to look around. You will be in awe to see that this is where the real you lives.

Another form of imagery is inner advisor imagery. Throughout history and in many religious traditions, people have sought the help of advisors. Native Americans speak of vision quests in which they travel alone into the wilderness for months at a time, awaiting advice from their spirit guides. This guide or vision gives the seeker important information and direction about his life's purpose. Others seek the advice of their guardian angels or their own spirit guides as part of their meditation practice. And what is prayer, other than requests for guidance and direction from a Divine Source, be it God, Jesus, Buddha or one's own Divine representation?

Are spirits real and available for our summoning? Does God answer our prayers? Do we have angels swarming about ready to help us for just the asking? Or are we just connecting to our own inner wisdom using these beings as imagery? I don't have the answers to these questions; but what I do know is guidance is always available. Whatever you choose to call it or where you believe it comes from, all you have to do is ask a question and guidance will follow.

You can think of inner advisor imagery as just another way of making your own inner guidance available to you, invariably bringing you closer to the real you. Call it your soul, Buddha nature, or that spark of the Divine that resides within each and every one of us.

Inner advisor meditation begins as all others, by closing your eyes, focusing on the breath, performing a brief body scan and image to bring you to a relaxed state. Then simply ask an advisor to appear. This can be a spirit, angel or a symbolic representation of your own inner voice, whose sole purpose is to help you understand who you are on a deeper level.

As with all other meditative practices, it is best to have no expectations. You may get an image of someone in your life, someone who has passed on, a being who represents your religious tradition, or someone you have never seen before. You may even sense an animal. Trying too hard engages your left brain in the process, which defeats the purpose. Accept whatever flashes before your mind's eye and consider whatever thoughts or feelings come up. Images that appear will come in momentary flashes; anything that takes longer may be tainted by conscious thought. I don't recommend taking action on any particular image until it is thoroughly contemplated and thought out. Giving your images respectful attention is all that is required.

A number of people/beings have shown up as inner advisors for me; but for reasons I don't understand, someone who looks like the Mona Lisa is my star player. I have no clue as to who this is supposed to symbolize for me. Perhaps the Virgin Mary, as Catholicism was an important part of my past. But then again, my Grandma Anna looked like the DaVinci masterpiece in her younger days. All I know is that whenever she appears in my mind's eye, I end up with insights otherwise unavailable.

If you have a regular prayer practice, this approach won't seem foreign; to others it may seem strange. What is important is that you have an open mind, don't second guess yourself, keep your intellect quiet, and be patient. The more relaxed and open you are, the more information you will get. The expectation of having mystical experiences will guarantee that they won't happen; so just relax and be open.

I can't stress enough that after any meditation in which you ask a question or contemplate a problem, with or without imagery, answers and information will come one way or another. Once you have engaged your subconscious mind, information will come to you in dreams, random flashes of insight, something you hear on TV, read in a book or magazine that you randomly pick up, and from other people. Pay particular attention to coincidences, which are jam-packed with meaning, but will notice only if you are paying attention. Just asking the question guarantees an answer at some point, though it may present itself in a way that you don't necessarily expect.

Active, Receptive, Inner Advisor Meditation
CD #1, Track #8
Music licensed through Megatrax Production Music, Inc.

Finally, imagery can be used to help you manifest your destiny. There is evidence to suggest that goals are more likely to be attained when you spend time imaging yourself successfully achieving whatever it is you desire. Writing down your short and long term goals in a journal is also a useful exercise. This gives them concrete expression and clearly states your intention. Without committing to a serious intention, goals can just float around in your own little fantasyland and are much less likely to come to fruition. If you add brief daily images of successful goal accomplishments to your daily meditation practice, you will have a powerful practice which I am certain will amaze you.

CHAPTER EIGHT

Lovingkindness

Lovingkindness and Tonglen are Buddhist meditations that help us tap into that part of our being which is capable of unconditional love. By means of sending love to ourselves, our loved ones, our enemies and sentient beings everywhere, we practice being more unconditionally loving and we increase our capacity for forgiveness and compassion. This meditative focus, used on a regular basis, benefits all of our relationships and opens our hearts to beings everywhere. A world in which this philosophy is practiced and embraced would be wonderful and peaceful. But the place to start is within yourself.

Being loving to and making peace with people in your life will make your relationships more satisfying; healing every part of your being invariably follows. I cannot think of a better way to help a person who is at the end of his/her life finish unfinished business; making for a peaceful transition. This practice was crucial for Lynn, as working through difficulties in some of her relationships was her only hope for a peaceful passing.

Lovingkindness is a meditation that focuses our attention on sending love to ourselves and others. No one could disagree that promoting love in the world has no downside, perhaps with the exception of my hero, Woody Allen, who mirrors our collective neuroses in the following quote:

> *To love is to suffer*
> *To avoid suffering, one must not love.*
> *But then one suffers from not loving.*
> *So to love is to suffer, not to love is to suffer, to suffer is to suffer*
> *To be happy is to love*
> *To be happy then is to suffer*
> *But suffering makes one unhappy.*
> *Therefore, to be unhappy, one must love or love to suffer*

LOVINGKINDNESS

Or suffer from too much happiness[1]

Unknowingly, Woody Allen is actually describing a Buddhist philosophy. This statement is an accurate description of love as we have come to know it; that is, love that is conditional and painful because of our attachment to some concept of the way it should be. The kind of love practiced in Lovingkindness and Tonglen meditation is described very nicely by Thich Nhat Hanh. "Happiness is only possible with true love. True love has the power to heal and transform the situation around us and bring a deep meaning to our lives." True love in this case refers to love, freely given, with no expectation of return and no attachment to its turning out in any particular way.

I can think of no example that makes the concept of unconditional love as clear as Mother Teresa. Leaving her comfortable convent to devote her life to picking up horribly infected and dying people off the street, pulling babies out of dumpsters just so that they can die in an environment of love and dignity is unconditional love in its most perfect form. When asked why she devoted so much time to people who had no hope of cure she answered simply that "just to love them is enough."

Every religion has this type of love as its foundation, as beautifully stated in Corinthians. "Though I speak in the tongues of man and angels but have not love, I am as sounding brass or a clanging cymbal, and though I have the gift of prophesy and understand all mysteries and all knowledge, and though I have all faith so as to move mountains but have not love, I am nothing."[2]

Over time, wars and disputes have been fought in the name of religion. This is quite an indictment of the human capacity to use whatever means possible to justify his actions. But when all is said and done, love is the true basis of all religions. Think what a different world this would be if we could live according to the principles on which we agree rather than kill each other over our differences. The Christian precept of "loving one's neighbor as oneself", so easy to say, not so easy to do, pales in comparison to the instruction that you should "love your enemies and pray for those who persecute you." Here we enter a realm that is foreign and almost impossible for the vast majority of us to put into practice.

If there is any religious philosophy that embraces and practices "love your enemy" it would have to be Buddhism, in which one vows to cause no harm to any sentient being, not even an insect, much less another human being; refusing to raise even a hand in war even when being attacked. Buddhists believe that "Whatever happiness is in the world has arisen from a wish for the welfare of others. Whatever misery there is arises from indulging in selfishness."[3]

Judaism teaches that loving and caring for others should be one's primary goal in life, as in this tradition, love of God means loving oneself and others. The word "Mitzvah" means kindness for its own sake. The Mitzvah of Tzedakah is the moral obligation to love and help those in need.[4]

Love and care for one another are central to a person's life purpose even in the much maligned Islamic religion. According to the Koran, "Paradise is for those who love one another, sit together and visit one another for God's sake."[5]

Lovingkindness and Tonglen are based on the Hindu Brahma-viharas, the belief that in order to enter the kingdom of heaven, to be with Brahma (God), one must practice and live a life based on unconditional love, compassion, and sympathetic joy (the ability to take joy in the good fortune of others). A person's willingness to embrace these principles also insures a life of equanimity; peace unshakable by the suffering inherent in human existence.

Heavenly aspirations aside, what does lovingkindness do for us mortals here and now? If practiced as a part of daily meditation, one's tendency toward loving unconditionally and feeling compassion toward others will increase. Your own happiness and the happiness of everyone you touch can't help but follow this core change in attitude and approach to life.

There are many kinds of love, but which types of love are in actuality unconditional? For those of you who were around in the late sixties and early seventies, love took on a different flavor than in times prior. The hippy concept of peace and love for everyone was very sweet, almost giving those of us who were involved the sense that a peaceful utopia might actually be possible in our lifetime. Naïve though it may have been, passing out flowers, greeting one another with the sign of peace, and protesting the war in Vietnam gave this generation hope that things could be different. But, the world, being what it was (and is) wasn't ready to embrace all that living this philosophy would entail. Walking the walk in this case would require the willingness of all of civilization to share equally in resources, let go of all need for power and control and accept once and for all that we are all One; another's happiness is our happiness. Unfortunately, we are nowhere near this ideal. Even the hippy movement deteriorated into sex, drugs, and rock and roll, signaling the end of an innocent and touching era.

Lovingkindness (or "metta" in Sanskrit) meditation is a practice which brings us closer to understanding the concept of the oneness of all things. Our willingness to send unconditional love to others, regardless of our relationship to them, helps us to see and feel our connection to everyone. Until this is accomplished, world peace is a term of value only to an aspiring Miss America. The only kind of love which brings true joy and promises peace is love given with no strings attached, no expectations, no clinging, and no grasping, therefore causing no suffering—the Mother Teresa kind of love.

Does this kind of love exist in nature? The image of my three dogs comes to mind. I have yet to meet a dog that doesn't show this kind of love better than any human I know. Dogs are always there, they love you no matter what, and their affection is there just for the asking. Aside from the necessities of food, water and rest, loving his family is more than adequate to his life's purpose.

What about your best, most trusted and beloved friend? We have all had the privilege of knowing a person with whom we can share anything, who won't abandon us no matter what, to whom we can go anytime, anywhere, for anything. This is someone who provides comfort and refuge when necessary; someone who is equally capable of reveling in our successes and mourning our sorrows. To me, this is about as close to unconditional love as it gets.

Do partners and family constitute love of the unconditional kind? There is no question that these are the people whom we should love unconditionally. Yet, in some ways, these relationships are where we encounter the most difficulty. The very nature of family relationships is bound up with conditions. We need to count on one another, we have expectations that our spouses, children and parents will behave a certain way, we have goals for them; and they have expectations of us. Thus, the very nature of our relationships with family members is one of expectation and attachment. It is not always easy to let go of our expectations and accept and love them for exactly who they are, yet this is what unconditional love demands.

For me, this is the best use of lovingkindness meditation. Family life can be full of turmoil, chaos, disagreements and disappointments. But we get into trouble when we can see nothing else and one angry encounter runs mindlessly into the next. Taking 5 or 10 minutes each day imaging your loved ones, focusing on their good qualities rather than obsessing about the bad, and sending them your loving best wishes can turn things around. My meditation cannot magically transform my teenage children into perfect little angels, but it opens and softens me toward them, and that makes all the difference. So no matter what transpires while everyone is running around in the morning, stressing over school, work, or whatever, taking time to focus on how much I love them allows me to come back again, punctuating all the pain and suffering with openness and love. It is not only a practice of letting go of our need to be right and accepting and loving others just as they are, but also of accepting our own imperfection.

In this culture, passion and love are often considered synonymous, but is there anything unconditional about passion? Passion is desire, wanting, needing, even to the point of the possession of the beloved. But passion, though romantic, fun and necessary for the propagation of the species, is cloaked in condition. Our expectation that exciting raw passion should continue unabated forever is why many marriages end in divorce. Equating love with passion sets one up for disappointment as one relationship after another self-destructs when passion, always a fleeting phenomenon, diminishes.

Long lasting happiness is impossible without the more mature view that love is a constantly changing emotion, of which passion is only a part. The Dalai Lama makes an astute point when he says, "Unlike those relationships based on caring and genuine affection, the pursuit of romantic love is based on fantasy, unattainable and likely to be a source of frustration."

So in lovingkindness meditation, we are sending love of the

unconditional kind first to ourselves and then to others. As with all meditation, this gives us repeated chances at practicing being unconditionally loving to everyone. The return on this investment of time is an ever-increasing understanding of our ultimate connectedness to everyone. Once realized, there is less need to be angry, jealous, fearful, selfish, or hostile because of an inner certainty that another person's happiness, sorrow, joy and suffering is our own.

In the *Dhammapada*, Buddha says, "Love can uproot fear, anger, guilt, it can go anywhere, no external condition can prevent it and no one and nothing can stop it." A child's fear of "the things that go bump in the night" vanishes when a loving parent appears with a hug. One cannot maintain an angry posture when true love is the foundation of a relationship. Guilt cannot survive when you know with certainty that the other, no matter what, loves you. Unconditional love is the one thing over which we have total dominion and is the only thing with the power to change the world.

To demonstrate this point I will share with you a Buddhist folk tale that describes how the practice of lovingkindness meditation helps to overcome fear. In this story, the Buddha's monks were sent into the forest to meditate for many weeks at a time. In the forest, they came across many frightening creatures and tree spirits. So fearful were they that they couldn't continue their practice. Learning this, the Buddha taught them to send lovingkindness to all of the things that frightened them, upon which every forest beast became loving and protective. This tale points out that our ability to cultivate a loving core not only affects our perceptions and our own sense of well-being, but will in fact influence everyone and everything that we touch personally or even in thought.

Peace Pilgrim was a woman who lived and exemplified this philosophy. At the age of 50, Peace Pilgrim abandoned her original identity and life with the purpose of working for world peace. She vowed that she would walk back and forth across the country until all parts of the world were no longer in conflict. Giving up all possessions, attired in sweat clothes and sneakers, she walked, stopping in communities to lecture on the need for global love and compassion. Living as a vagrant, sleeping under bridges and the like, accepting food and shelter only when offered, she never had a moment's fear, as her love for all of humankind was so great, she simply couldn't conceive of being threatened by another being.

A man who met Peace Pilgrim along the way had his life change forever. As he tells the story, he was an addicted vagrant, admittedly not a very nice person. One night, when seeing her sleeping under a bridge, he went over to her with the intention of raping or even murdering her. As he approached, she greeted him with a warm smile saying, "Oh, I am so glad that you are here. With you beside me, I know I will be safe," then fell into a peaceful sleep. At this moment, the man's life was forever changed by nothing more than the strength of her unconditional love.

Peace Pilgrim continued to walk, traversing the country some 30 times until her death at some time in her eighties. Her philosophies are beautifully preserved in a number of books published by an organization bearing her name.

According to the Buddha, benefits of lovingkindness meditation include an increased ability to sleep and have pleasant dreams. It promises that humans, animals and celestial beings will love and protect you. You will never be harmed by any external danger. You will be radiant and peaceful in life and at death you will be unconfused and have the promise of being reborn in happy realms. The biblical concept, "As we sow, so shall we reap," is in total harmony with the eastern concept of karma, recognizing that each and every one of our actions will have a consequence. When you greet the world with love and compassion, it will be returned to you many times over. And have no doubt that anger, distrust and hatred will behave similarly. The Dalai Lama says, "My religion is kindness." Imagine what this world would be like if all religions felt this way.

Joan Borysenko says, "The best measure of a full life is not in its length, but in its love." As I watched hundreds of people filing in to my friend Lynn's memorial service, it was clear that even though she was only 40 at the time of her death, her life was very full. There wasn't a person there who didn't have a story about the impact that her love, generosity and caring had on his or her life. Always freely, quietly and thoughtfully given, her love was subtle and true, affecting each and every one of us on a deep level.

Thomas Merton, a Trappist monk, contemplated the qualities

that make a person a saint. He writes, "Sanctity is not what's important, it is their ability to see the beauty in another—to admire everyone else. They have the clarity of compassion that can find the good in every being—the eagle in the egg, the butterfly in the caterpillar and the beauty in the sinner."

"Namaste", the Hindu word used both to greet to say good-bye, sets one's intention to always look for the very best in a person. It means I bow to the God like part of you or I recognize your Buddha within. Eastern traditions are based on the assumption that every sentient being is basically good and loving. Our responsibility is to recognize a person's true goodness as a way of helping him discover it within himself. Lovingkindness meditation encourages us to see the best in others, to recognize the best part of ourselves, and encourage others to do the same. Mother Teresa saw Jesus in every person that she cared for and understood that "any act of love is a work of peace, no matter how small."

Compassion, the second of the Hindu Brahma-viharas is the wish and the ability to relieve the suffering of others. One's ability to feel true compassion is a real gift to bring to a therapeutic relationship, as there is no trait more likely to promote healing. Western medical education is unsurpassed in teaching the medical knowledge and technical skill needed for curing physical illness, but it is compassion that heals.

When one is treating a small child in pain, compassion is easy to come by. However, in an ER setting, there are often people walking through the door for whom compassionate treatment is difficult at best. "Bleeding heart" is a term used by some to describe those who can treat even the disenfranchised compassionately, as if this represents a weakness of some sort. Neither strength nor weakness, compassion is nothing more than one's attempt to see what may have given rise to a person's situation and to understand what it must be like to live as he/she does. Despite the inability to change a person's situation, compassionate care is never wasted, as I believe that even the most difficult patient will benefit from it on some level. Feeling compassion for our patients helps us as well. Having disdain for the drug addict, alcoholic or the delinquent child hurts the worker more than the patient. It denigrates the value of his or her chosen vocation and ultimately one's self.

Compassion allows us to look at difficult people and their problems as a response to unfortunate conditions in their lives. Henry Wadsworth Longfellow wrote, "If we could read the secret history of our enemies, we should find in each man's life sorrow and suffering to disarm all hostility."[6] Compassion does not mean condoning someone's destructive behavior nor does it mean that one should bring every drug addict home in the futile attempt to save him. Compassion is simply an attempt to understand and accept the person, just as he or she is. To judge that individual is detrimental to both parties. According to Buddha, "Compassion helps us to learn to have sympathy for all beings without exception." The person whom this ultimately benefits the most is oneself.

So, one may ask, what's in it for me? As part of one's role in health care or simply being a friend, compassion does more for the person doing the supporting than it does for the one needing support. Lynn's allowing me into her life during her illness and dying process was the best gift she could give me. The compassion I felt for her touched me so deeply and opened me so completely that my life will never be the same. Her questions began my own search into the meaning of life; her needs made me realize that only by reaching into the depths of my own heart and soul could I be of any real help to her and ultimately to myself. As a result, my own growth has been immeasurable.

In a 30-year study of Harvard graduates, George Vaillant learned that an altruistic lifestyle is one of the prime indicators of good mental health. In another study of several thousand people, Allan Luks found that 90 percent of people who volunteer their time and resources for causes they care about report a "high" associated with these activities. In general, volunteers appear to be more peaceful and calm than non-volunteers, demonstrate an increased sense of self-worth and tend to have fewer stress-related disorders. James House, from the University of Michigan Research Center, discovered that volunteers also enjoy increased vitality and lived longer.[7]

Mr. and Mrs. Bell, a lovely couple in their seventies volunteer regularly in my emergency room. They are the most vibrantly happy, glowing people I have had the pleasure to meet. Not only do they lend support to patients who are sick and in pain, but they always have candy to for the employees. Something so simple has such far reaching benefits as each person they touch smiles, softens and in one way or another will pass this kindness on. Mr. and Mrs. Bell have no concept of their contribution and really don't need to; as the act itself surely does as much for them as it does for everyone they touch.

Sir John Templeton has invested a great deal of his enormous wealth into research that studies the effect of spirituality on health and well-being. He feels that joy naturally follows one's willingness to bring happiness to others. "People devote much time and energy to seeking happiness, but the sad fact is that we are often seeking it outside ourselves. Actually, the happiest people are those who are working to give happiness to others. Happiness is not found by seeking it; it is a by-product of caring about other people."[8]

One does not have to be a millionaire or even in good circumstances to show this generosity of spirit. Victor Frankl, a Holocaust survivor, in his book *Man's Search for Meaning,* discusses his observation that there were certain individuals who not only survived, but actually thrived while living in concentration camps. "We who lived in the concentration camps can remember those who walked through the huts comforting others, giving away their last piece of bread…They may have been few in number, but they offer sufficient proof that everything can be taken from us but the last of human freedoms…the freedom to *choose* one's attitude in any circumstance."[9] The survivors of this unspeakable horror were those who chose to find meaning in loving generosity and compassion for others. "The freedom to choose attitude in any circumstance …" choice, no matter what, we always have choice.

One would think that a mathematical genius the caliber of Albert Einstein would be solely left-brained and that the suffering of the human race would be of little consequence to him. In truth, he claims that most of his theories came to him in strokes of right-brained intuition. It was this very same brilliant intuition that convinced him of the interdependence of all things and the necessity for each of us to live lives of compassion. "We become imprisoned and blinded by our thoughts and feelings because they are conceived only with our lives and desires as separate beings. Our experience of ourselves as separate and enduring is a delusion and ultimately imprisoning. If we never come to know that part of us that is whole, we only see one side of being alive. We need to intentionally cultivate compassion for all of life, an appreciation of ourselves and all living creatures. This work is intrinsically healing."

So, what's in it for me? Pure joy. Living a loving and compassionate life promises joy to ourselves and everyone we touch. The human quest for happiness need not go any further than developing the capacity to love unconditionally and meeting the world with compassion. And understanding again and again that everything we need is right here where we are, in this moment.

The third of the Brahma viharas is sympathetic joy. This is the ability to feel joy for the happiness of others. Happiness about our own good fortune couldn't be easier; however, it becomes difficult when it is someone else who is finding success, winning the lottery or getting the man of her dreams. Jealousy, envy, comparing, competition and prejudice are just a few of the many states that get in the way of our feeling happy for someone else. It is almost as if there is a finite amount of good stuff to be had and if someone else gets it, we won't. The truth is that joy and love are infinite; there is plenty to go around. Love breeds more love, and joy breeds more joy. The more you give, the more you get. Your ability to be generous, loving and joyful about another's good fortune will come back to you many times over.

Gratitude for the blessings in one's own life is a prerequisite for the ability to feel sympathetic joy. When one is grateful for what he has, his own wellspring of happiness is filled to the brim. Feeling joy for others naturally follows as a bubbling over of this sense of abundance. On the other hand, a person who goes through life never having enough, always grasping for what he/she doesn't have rather than recognizing what he does, is likely to be envious and angry toward anyone and everyone who has something that he doesn't. Without a drastic change in attitude, this person has no chance of finding happiness that is anything but a short- lived, fleeting response to some material gain.

Interdependence, the inner knowing that all beings are intimately connected, leads directly to one's ability to feel sympathetic joy. Any person who touches this reality understands that one's own and another's happiness are one and the same. Lovingkindness meditation is a practice that ultimately helps a person experience this state on a deep level, helping her to derive pleasure from another's good fortune, while compounding her own joy.

Equanimity, the final Brahma vihara, is a quality of unshakable inner peace. Like Mount Everest which stands unchangeable, whether under sunshine, clouds, ice or storm, a person with equanimity has a peaceful core, steadfast, no matter what turmoil may be raging all around. The ability to pull oneself out of the chaos, to settle down into a silent witnessing of his life through the window of the right brain is the promise of meditation. Once recognized, this core of tranquility can be accessed at will. By helping us to view our lives and our world through the window of unconditional love, lovingkindness meditation brings a profound sense of peace. Stated beautifully by Sharon Salzberg, "A loving mind can meet peace and joy one moment, grief the next and not be shattered by the change."

She also said, "The greatest gift we can offer to the world is our own peaceful heart."[10] How does "one's own peaceful heart" affect others? Lovingkindness meditation affects those around us both directly and indirectly. Indirectly, when you consciously set out to make your attitudes more loving, loving actions will follow. Others can't help but respond positively to actions that are fueled by love.

More inconceivable, perhaps, is the idea that lovingkindness meditation may actually affect people directly even if there is no actual contact with that person. Some studies have suggested that some part of an individual's consciousness can extend beyond his own body and actually influence those for whom the meditation was intended. This phenomenon, known as non-local mind, will be discussed at length in Chapter 12. But for now, simply remain open to the possibility.

My first experience of this phenomenon occurred several years ago when I attended a conference during which I learned and practiced lovingkindness meditation. Once in a fully relaxed state, we were instructed to send our loving wishes using the image of a beautiful healing light to the people in our lives. I got so emotionally involved with this exercise, that flowing tears added to an intense euphoria. Eventually returning to left-brain mode, the memory of the experience faded. When I got home, I was stunned when my teenage daughter who, despite being at an age where mothers are best neither seen nor heard, met me on the stairway with, "Mom, I don't know why, but I missed you so much today. I love you so much." Even my adolescent son, who would generally greet me with a grunt, offered a hug, followed by my younger daughter, energetically bouncing down to get in on the action. Finally, my husband whose focus on whatever computer project he is working on generally wins any competition between it and me, also greeted me with the whole family on the stairs. Coincidence you say? Perhaps; but suffice it to say, it got my attention.

Quasi-scientist that I am, I thought I would try an informal study. While walking on the beach over the course of several weeks, I would randomly choose people from a distance to whom I would send lovingkindness meditation; call them Group 1. Those in Group 2 experienced only my passing presence. In the vast majority of cases, those to whom I sent my silent, loving best wishes acknowledged me with a huge smile, going out of their way to say "hello," while most of Group 2 walked by without any acknowledgement. OK, so this isn't the air tight study design that would be accepted by the New England Journal of Medicine, but it does suggest an interesting trend.

One such day I was in such a state of bliss, I was totally unaware of going 70 in a 40-mile-per-hour zone, wherein a local police officer appropriately summoned me over to the side of the road. Normally, the sight of blue flashing lights in the rear view mirror would plunge me into left-brain reality; but not this time. Anyway, now sending loving wishes to the officer, his family and everyone he's ever met, I greet him with license, registration and an ecstatic grin, the equivalent of one that might be seen on a newly brainwashed cult member. After checking the documents, the officer said, "Mrs. Johnson, I won't give you a ticket, but the reason I stopped you is I am concerned about you and I don't want you to get hurt." Driving away I wondered, is it possible that my loving intentions actually made a change in this police officer's demeanor? Or, was it the fact that I was twice his age, a speeding cute little old lady of no real danger to anyone? Who knows?

Whatever the reason I got out of a well-deserved speeding ticket, this experience illustrates the point that a loving attitude can change one's view of and how one is perceived in the world.

Remember, meditation is something that is done for its own sake, for what it does for your inner being, and would not be useful or effective as a means of mind control nor as a practice to be used to get out of speeding tickets!

There is a lot of literature suggesting that anything which encourages one's loving attitudes will have a positive effect on his/her health. All systems of the human body are positively influenced by love, the practice of compassion, and how connected we feel to ourselves and others. Studies of women in breast cancer support groups, all other treatments being equal, have shown that their life expectancy is twice as long as those not participating.[11]

We have already seen that meditation improves one's immune system. But lovingkindness in particular has compelling effects. Meditation increases saliva IgA, a measurable indicator of strong immune function, but it is increased even further when fueled by loving intention. A study done with students demonstrated that IgA levels are universally higher in students whose primary motive in life is friendship than in those who valued competition and power above all else.[12]

An interesting, though admittedly quirky, study was done in which volunteers were asked to spit into a cup before and after being in a room where a film of Mother Teresa was being shown. The supposition was that people would feel more loving and generous because of being in her presence. The experimenters were interested in learning whether this would translate into increased immune function. What they discovered was saliva IgA was markedly elevated in the post-lecture sputum and remained elevated for a few weeks after.[13]

Overall, research has indicated that love or social support is a better predictor of good health than any other health choice, including diet and exercise. Epidemiologists were particularly interested in a community called Roseto, in which there was a remarkably low incidence of coronary artery disease. Expecting to find people who were super health conscious, they were surprised to discover that their diets were, if anything, less healthy than the average. There was a high incidence of smoking and a population that was not particularly physically fit. The only distinguishing feature of this place was the fact that the townspeople were close knit, took care of one another, celebrated and mourned together. Social connection seemed to be the variable responsible for the remarkable lack of heart disease.[14]

Single, widowed and divorced smoking males are at greatest risk for heart disease. Although we tend to see smoking as the real cardiac bad guy, an interesting observation showed that married smokers and divorced non-smokers have the same rate of heart disease. So a non-smoking male who isn't in a relationship has the same risk of developing coronary artery disease as a married smoker. Therefore, most would agree that for men, marriage is a healthy lifestyle, unless you believe as an acquaintance of Dr. Bernie Siegel who said, "So, if you want to die a slow and lingering death, get married."

Studies have shown that loneliness predisposes people to a number of conditions. In one study, females who reported feeling lonely, due to difficult or abusive relationships, have a 2.4 times greater risk of hormone-related malignancies, specifically breast and ovarian cancer. This probably comes as no surprise. What did surprise me, however, was that those with few or no social contacts have a risk 5 times the normal. So being in a fulfilling relationship has clearly been shown to be beneficial to your health. Bernie Siegel sums this up by saying, "When you have your health, you do not have everything, but when you don't have your health but do have people who care for you and love you, you do have everything."

Finally, one of my favorite studies is one done by Robert Nerem, in which rabbits were given high cholesterol diets to see how long it would take for them to develop heart disease. As the experimenters regularly measured cholesterol levels, they kept getting data that they found confusing. Apparently only the bunnies in the top row of cages actually developed hypercholesterolemia, while those in the lower rows did not. It turned out that the petite lab tech could only reach the rabbits in the lower rows; so it was only these bunnies she played and snuggled with everyday. Those in the top row just had their food pushed into the bottom of their cages. [15] Additional studies were done using physical affection as the variable with the same results.

When all is said and done, loving connection has benefits not only to humans, but to animals as well. Perhaps the Buddhists are right—that we are connected in some inexplicable way to all sentient beings, and should therefore treat them as we ourselves would like to be treated.

Formal lovingkindness meditation is one in which you mentally send your love and best wishes to various people in your life. The traditional Buddhist practice starts by sending these messages first to yourself, then to a benefactor, loved ones and families, neutral persons and finally even to your enemies or difficult persons in your life. In formal practice, one uses formal phrases, similar to a mantra such as, "May you be well, may you be happy, may you be healthy, may you be filled with lovingkindness and may you be at peace."

Although we don't generally think of sending kind, loving wishes to ourselves, this is where you must start, as the quality of love that you send to others will only be as good as the extent to which you are able to see the value of and love yourself. Unfortunately, we tend focus on those things we don't like about ourselves. We are never smart, thin, attractive, or rich enough. Unless our own cup is full to the brim, there isn't enough left over to give to others. The practice of self-lovingkindness is one in which you consciously look at the goodness in yourself. Appreciate your generosity and the kind deeds you have done. Give yourself credit for your successes; it doesn't have to be anything earth shattering. Sometimes just getting through a difficult situation can be a major success for which you deserve enormous credit. When you take a few moments to appreciate yourself, you can't help but feel more joy. This is the essential foundation for being able to offer genuine love to others.

Self-lovingkindness also requires that you look at your imperfections, but not in a demeaning way. Look at your anger, guilt, addictions and mistakes and surround these parts of yourself with compassion and lovingkindness. Use phrases such as, "May I accept these things, may I be gentle with myself, may I learn to love myself not only despite these things, but because of my ability to endure them. May these difficulties help me to feel compassion for others in a similar circumstance." Imperfection is part of being human; grace comes along with compassionate and loving acceptance of everything that we are. As we begin to view ourselves in a more positive light, our worldview changes accordingly.

The next instruction is to send lovingkindness to your

benefactor. This is a person in your past or present who has loved you unconditionally. This may be someone who has given you encouragement, or has been generous with his/her spirit. This is a person for whom you feel respect, love and gratitude, to whom sending loving wishes is effortless. My benefactor is the most caring and loving physician I have had the privilege to know. Without him, I would never have thought myself good or smart enough to even consider becoming a physician. I don't know of anything that has honored me more than his heartfelt belief that I could walk in his footsteps. There is no one for whom sending loving best wishes comes more naturally. In your mind's eye, picture one or more such people; recall the many ways in which they have helped you and bask in their goodness. Then send your wishes: "May you be well, may you be happy, may you be at peace, may your life be filled with lovingkindness."

Lovingkindness, per tradition, is then sent to beloved friends. Picture this person; consider what this friendship means to you; think about the qualities in this person that are worthy of admiration. Ponder those times that he/she was there for you, supporting you through difficult times, celebrating with you through the good times. Thank him or her for not only her willingness but for her joy in being with you through darkness and light, thick and thin. With focused concentration, send him or her your loving best wishes.

The next category is the neutral person. The instruction here is to picture a person whom you see on a regular basis, but have never really spoken to—perhaps someone who works in your building or someone you see walking in the park; it could be anyone. It is fascinating to observe the changes in yourself and in the other person as you quietly send him loving messages day by day. You will find that your feelings toward him will grow to the extent that just seeing him will make you happy. As described in my beach experiment, observe also the changes that take place in the person for whom this meditation was intended. On some level, he or she will change as well. This is an amazing process, which shows that our loving intention toward others, even those we don't know, can be a powerful transformative practice.

Lisa was a student in the first workshop I taught. She came to class a week after the lovingkindness lecture with a huge smile and obvious excitement, with the news that her neutral person, someone who came to her office regularly for years who had never spoken to anyone, spoke to her. By the end of the week, Lisa's coworkers noticed that he was hanging around her desk, engaging in daily conversation. When they asked her what was going on, she told them she had been sending lovingkindness meditation to this man. Despite how improbable this may sound, try this yourself and be amazed.

Lovingkindness toward spouses or partners is in some ways a paradox. On the one hand, you love this person more than anybody else and as such, sending loving messages is effortless. However, these most intimate of relationships, by virtue of their intensity and importance to us, can at times, be a source of conflict and pain. Once again, the Buddhist concept of attachment (this being the relationship in which we are most attached) says that the level of our attachment is directly proportional to its potential to make us suffer. It is not the fact that we love these people but that we go into these relationships attached to the concept of living totally and blissfully happy ever after. The degree to which this is our expectation is the degree to which we will be sad, angry and disappointed when our (and our partner's) humanness with all its imperfections shows itself, as it invariably does.

The benefits of lovingkindness meditation here are twofold. First, on those days in which the relationship is blissful and a source of pleasure, focusing on how much you love this person is a source of great joy. But, on those days when there has been disagreement or conflict, your ability to get past whatever it is and choose instead to focus on those things that you love about him/her can't help but soften your attitude and make you consider what is really important. This is not to say that one should ever stay in a relationship that has become abusive or detrimental. In toxic relationships, the purpose of meditation is to help you see clearly enough to make whatever changes are in your own best interest. But what I am talking about here is that the practice of lovingkindness helps one to smooth out the rough edges. It gives you the ability to re-enter the relationship anew without cumulative carryover from one disagreement to the next.

The same thing applies to one's children. On the one hand, we love our children unconditionally, yet there is enormous guilt during those challenging times that are a part of every parent-child relationship. Although we truly love them, there are times, especially during the teenage years, when our sweet, loving babies act out in rebellious ways. Although this may be a necessary part of separating from us in preparation for separate adult lives, parents can't help but feel unloved and as though we have failed in our most important job.

Practicing lovingkindness meditation has been a lifesaver for my relationship with my children, especially during adolescence. Taking the time to settle down, hypnotize that trouble-making, fearful amygdala and left brain, and viewing them through my more loving, accepting, creative, spiritual right brain allows me to see our relationship in an entirely different light. I remember how very much I love them and how important it is to re-enter our relationship, time after difficult time, with a foundation of love and caring. When my teenage children and I are going at it, my ever-tranquil husband reminds me that I am the adult in the situation. As annoying as it is to hear this, he is right. As parents, it is our responsibility to do our best to set the tone for the best possible relationship with our children. This does not mean that we let them abuse us, let them run wild, or that we have no expectations from them; it means that we come back again and again, and punctuate the many conflicts with as much love and support as we can muster. For me, this is far and away the most valuable use of lovingkindness meditation. With my oldest child Anna, now age 22, I can see occasional glimpses of the light at the end of the tunnel. But with my youngest daughter now age 16, I will get a lot more practice, which, I guess, God help me, is a good thing.

It is important to find a way to remind one's child of his/her intrinsic goodness and beauty, especially during adolescence. Finding his or her personal identity is a scary process during which he or she is simultaneously a child and an adult, seeking freedom but requiring limits, needing closeness and distance, and craving your love while doing everything possible to test it. Your effort at being unconditionally loving can show your child that you recognize that underneath it all, there is a beautiful, loving spirit—"the eagle in the egg, the butterfly in the caterpillar and the beauty in the sinner."

Always remember the complicated nature of our most intimate relationships—we have expectations, we do need to count on one another, and we need to maintain some modicum of peaceful coexistence despite different needs and personalities. Unconditional love is critical but difficult. Our guilt doesn't help anyone. By first bathing yourself and then others in quiet, accepting, loving intention, you are giving it your best shot. No one can ask for anything more. Remember, we are human; this is very hard and you must be gentle with yourself. Nowhere is it more important to practice lovingkindness.

In summary, lovingkindness meditation and the attitudes that naturally follow soften your heart, help you to dissipate anger, and make you look at what is important. This can't help but change you and everyone you touch. You must face your feelings. Viewing your life in silence through the vision of your right brain accesses the very best part of yourself. Finally, when you *really* get the concept that another's bad behavior toward you comes from his/her own suffering, you have the possibility of truly caring for others.

Practicing lovingkindness meditation makes it a habit that makes you more likely to greet the world in a more loving way and brings you closer and closer to the ideal of unconditional love. Though this doesn't turn you into a doormat, justify someone's bad treatment of you, mean you should allow yourself to be hurt and make you deny your anger, it helps you to be more graceful in its expression. While you should not expect that this or any type of meditation will guarantee that nothing bad will ever happen, it will help you to meet whatever challenges present themselves with more equanimity.

This exercise demonstrates how your view of the world can change in a way that can't help but benefit yourself and everyone you touch simply by focusing on loving intention.

Formal Lovingkindness Meditation
CD 2, Track 1
Music licensed through Megatrax Production Music, Inc.

CHAPTER NINE

Forgiveness

The practice of sending lovinkindness not only to those we love but also to our enemies or difficult people is done to help us develop the quality of forgiveness. We generally think that forgiveness means letting someone who has done us harm off the hook. Forgiveness is actually the healthiest and most freeing choice that you can make for yourself. Holding resentment toward someone keeps you tied to him/her and to all the sadness and anger that defined that relationship. Mired in the negative past, you are unable to move on with what could be a happier life. When you are unable to forgive someone, your heart remains closed, not only to that person, but also to others with whom you may actually have a loving, fulfilling relationship. You cannot live a fulfilled life as long as you dwell and remain tied to someone else's harmful past actions. Therefore, forgiveness is the decision to let go of the past so that *you* can move on. But please be clear about this; it *does not* mean condoning someone else's bad behavior or allowing him or her back into your life.

Studies have shown that the ability to forgive has enormous health benefits. But the real gift of forgiveness is the inner peace that invariably comes along with it. No one claims that this is easy; in fact, it is the most difficult thing that you will have to do over and over again throughout your life.

I have sat with many people, including two of my best friends, at the end of their lives, and it has become clear that forgiveness at this time is without a doubt the most important thing that the dying person has to do. A person's chance to pass peacefully from here to whatever comes next is intimately tied to his ability to forgive himself and others. It is not unusual for a person nearing the end to look at all the ways he or she failed, could have done better and all the people he has hurt. This can cause a great deal of suffering. Hanging on to anger and resentment toward those who have caused them pain, only compounds their own pain. Therefore, forgiveness at the end of one's life allows the best possibility for a peaceful transition.

FORGIVENESS

There are various kinds and levels of forgiveness. Starting with examples of profound forgiveness may help to put this into a larger perspective. Jack Kornfield, an American trained as a Buddhist monk, speaks about the years following the Vietnam War in Cambodia when the dictator, Pol Pot, orchestrated the torture and murder of millions of Cambodians. Those who were "spared" had to face not only a life without their loved ones, but with hatred – the natural human response to such an atrocity. Some time after this, he and Maha Gosananda, a Cambodian monk, decided to hold a Buddhist ceremony to which all were invited. Having no idea how many would come, they may not have been prepared when some 10,000 people showed up.

So, what could one possibly say to help those people who had to endure such hatred and senseless violence? What could one say to heal a situation of this magnitude? Maha Gosananda said only this quote from the Buddha in the *Dhammapada*, "Hatred never ceases by hatred, but by love alone, is healed. This is an eternal law." Repeating this phrase over and over brought the entire gathering to tears. Essentially, he was asking these people to let go of their hatred and forgive the person who caused them indescribable suffering. They were not being asked to let Pol Pot off the hook, nor to condone his atrocities in any way, but to understand that when all is said and done, **hatred only hurts the person who hates**. Nothing could change what this vile dictator did. Being forgiven by the people he tortured was of no consequence to him. But what was important for the Cambodian people was the recognition that hatred kept them chained to past horror and served only to continue to deprive them of their own lives.

History has shown that there have been countless such unspeakable horrors in human history which as we know continue to this day. In the early fifties, when the Dalai Lama was a young man, the Chinese came into Tibet murdering and forcing the Tibetan people out of their own homes and country. Because Buddhists believe that defending oneself by harming another, even during war, is morally reprehensible, the Tibetans were tortured, murdered or forced to immigrate to India, where many still live to this day. Many Westerners consider this response to be a sign of weakness or cowardice. We are raised to believe that defending our way of life and protecting the rights of other endangered countries is not only a right but a moral

101

obligation. But when you really consider the sacrifice involved, the ability to stand up for one's principles and morality to this degree is strength beyond anything any of us have ever witnessed and is beyond our comprehension.

As much as I feel at the core of my being that they are right, how many of us would be able to watch the World Trade Center Towers fall and not feel as though clear, aggressive action would be justified? As much as I believe in this loving Buddhist philosophy if I were the President of the United States, I don't know what I would have done. Is it ever right to allow holocausts to happen?

Despite the fact the Dalai Lama and his followers have been exiled away from their homeland, they maintain a practice of daily prayers for the Chinese. Believing, as they do, that people would not be able to carry out such atrocious acts unless they were suffering horribly, they pray for an end to the suffering of the Chinese people. Though taking lovingkindness to a global level may seem unimaginable at this time in human history, one must start in one's own heart. The Bhagavad-Gita says, "If you want to see the brave, look at those who can forgive. If you want to see the heroic, look at those who can love in return for hatred." This statement is of course identical to the perhaps more familiar instruction of Judeo-Christian origin to... "Love your enemies and pray for those who persecute you."

So, should we forgive those who have done major harm in our lives? **YES**... Why? **Because Hatred Only Hurts You.** Does this mean that you need to allow this person in your life to abuse you even more? **ABSOLUTELY NOT!** It means only that you need to let go of the painful past and those associated with it so that you can move on with your *own* future. Forgiveness allows us to let go of the hurt, which serves only to increase *our own* suffering.

How does one begin this awesome process? Lovingkindness meditation is a great way to begin. It is important to start with those individuals, like teenage children, whom it is crucial to forgive. These relationships are central to whom we are and we must do whatever it takes to respond in as loving a way as is humanly possible.

Next, direct your lovingkindness meditation to minor enemies. These are those irritating folks whose presence in your life may not be as important as difficult loved ones, but whose annoying qualities and negative attitudes bring turmoil into your life. The Dalai Lama suggests that we think of these people as "opportunities to practice patience."

A participant in one of my classes returned a few weeks after beginning her lovingkindness practice beaming with the news that her husband's angry ex-wife spoke to her for the first time in years. By the end of their conversation, there was no doubt that a friendly, caring, connection, had been made. Is it possible that these unpleasant situations and people can be turned around using nothing more than your loving intention? Try it, you have nothing to lose.

Finally, as you practice and get more comfortable with this approach to conflict, start working on the major difficult people in your life. Embrace the notion that someone's bad behavior toward you is there for one reason and one reason only — his own suffering. If you look deeply at people who have done you harm, you will see pain. And though this in no way justifies his/her behavior, it might make it a little easier to look past his actions and find some miniscule part of him that is good. Namaste—look for that divine spark, for that elusive Buddha nature within him or her, however deeply buried.

Opening your heart in this way does not mean that you will open the door and let this person hurt you again. It is simply your attempt to let go of all the hurt so that you can carry on with your life. Lovingkindness meditation for difficult people in our lives keeps them in our hearts, yet does not allow them to continue to hurt us. Closing your heart to one person guarantees that you will not fully be able to open it to others. Don't let anyone take away your own potential for love.

How is it possible to get to the point where you can do lovingkindness meditation on behalf of the bad actors, the child abusers, rapists, and murderers? Or should you? Yes, no better or worse, perhaps, than Pol Pot, they do need to be forgiven, for *your* sake. You must start this process first by feeling compassion for yourself. Without a doubt, there is a time for grieving, a time for anger and a time for licking one's wounds, but the time also comes to let go and move on.

Lovingkindness to enemies is a practice where you try to

separate the person from the act and attempt to find that part of him/her which is good. Pema Chodron says, even if you have to picture what he was like as an infant, it provides a starting point. If you can't manage any of this, simply recognize his wish to be happy. Wish him an end to the suffering that has made him the person that he is. The more you practice with this, the fewer enemies you will have. This is the ultimate goal for your own health and well-being,

Let me tell you about Claire, the person who has taught me about the need for forgiveness. Claire was my mom, an alcoholic, and one of the saddest people I have ever known. Not unlike most alcoholics, she was abusive, not physically, not in the "Mommie Dearest," sense, but in unpredictable, subtle ways so characteristic of addicted personalities. Being particularly skilled at making one feel guilty rather than angry, alcoholics have a way of making those around them, particularly their children, feel responsible for the pervasive unhappiness. She had an emptiness that could never be filled, only numbed by alcohol and Valium. Her hostility, covered by an adequate veneer of sweetness when necessary, was the result of a primitive anger at everyone for not having the ability to make her happy. Although she could be loving, fun and generous at times, especially when in plain view of people outside of the family, alcohol brought out a manipulative mean spiritedness, which I now realize was a more tolerable way for her to express the depth of sorrow, which was her true reality.

What self-esteem my mom had was intimately connected to physical symptoms and illness, real or imagined. These things temporarily gave her the attention for which she yearned. When her own symptoms were inadequate, she quickly latched on to any minor, ordinary complaints that I had and turned them into life threatening dramas. As a child desperate to do anything to make my mom happy, I spent many a day submitting to unnecessary medical testing, procedures and hospital admissions, giving her only a momentary reason for being.

Swinging from self-loathing to martyrdom, from caring for to needing to be taken care of, from a bright, vivacious public persona to a needy, intoxicated, behind closed doors neurotic, my mom wasn't different from any number of people with alcohol addiction. Nor was I any different from other children whose lives were confused at best and well, much worse at worst. In this situation, with not so subtle assistance from the parent, the child learns that he/she is never good enough, having failed in his/her first and most important goal – making Mom happy. Never knowing what is coming next, the child responds either by becoming super responsible or by following the parent right into the downward spiral. By the grace of God, I chose the former. Living in hope that the good times will last and dying in despair, each time they don't, the child of the alcoholic vows "next time I will be better, next time I will try harder and one day, my mom will be happy." But the truth is, no matter what the child does, she can never be good enough and the sadness lingers. No matter what we do, the alcoholic's unfathomable emptiness remains unfilled.

As a child, one has neither the experience nor the vocabulary to help him or her get a handle on what is going on, but the desire for the ideal family never ceases. Years later, when the light dawns that your parent is an alcoholic, despite now having both the word and the experience, the yearning persists. And later still, even armed with clinical psychology training, and the stunning diagnoses of Munchausen's disease (the need to be physically ill for its secondary gain) and Munchausen's by proxy (the need to have one's child ill for the mother's secondary gain), the pain, loss and disappointment continue, unremitting.

With education and the sophistication that follows, forgiveness of one's parents is an intellectual forgone conclusion. After all, I was a psychiatric social worker at that time, and if I couldn't forgive someone who was emotionally disabled, then who could? But what I have come to realize is that intellectual and emotional forgiveness are entirely different animals. Intellectually, I was done with this by my mid–twenties, but emotionally, not until I was near 50, a few months before her death.

What makes heart felt forgiveness so difficult? No matter how old one gets, there is always the hope that the idealized parent for whom you have always yearned will somehow miraculously rise from the ashes. Yet time after disappointing time, it doesn't happen; the parent remains just who he or she is regardless of your wishes. But the bigger fear is that if you allow forgiveness to open your heart, you will get hurt again and again. Persistent anger or resentment toward the parent sets up an impenetrable wall whose sole function is to keep that little child who continues to live inside of you safe, though imprisoned on some level.

Lovingkindness meditation practice has helped me immeasurably in giving me a way to look deeply into my mother's history of suffering, which I am certain was significant. Having spent almost a year of her babyhood in the hospital for a kidney condition and being an only child, my mother's parents unwittingly treated her like an invalid from the beginning. It therefore makes sense that she would continue to equate love and attention with illness and symptoms. Caring for a sick child is the only kind of mothering she understood; therefore, her ability to love and mother me was somewhat dependent on her perception that I was ill, though this was never the case in actuality.

Understanding that any harm done to me was unintentional and completely unconscious, I am able to look beyond her unskillful actions and get occasional glimpses of the parts of her, which were good and kind.

I also came to realize that without her being exactly who she was, I wouldn't be exactly who I am. Since I have grown to like and respect the person that I am, I'd have to say it was worth whatever it took to get me here. Having let go of my need for her to measure up to my expectations, I am free to see the best parts of her and am no longer imprisoned by the scary parts. Finally, and perhaps most importantly, I have come to realize that she, without a doubt, did the very best that she could; *everyone does.*

A few weeks before my mom died, I had the opportunity to share all of this with her—a brief life review, if you will, of our time together in this lifetime. As I spoke to her, a sweet, beatific, smile emerged from her own place of stillness. Wordlessly, in that precious moment, I glimpsed that Buddha nature of which I have read, spoken and written so many times. A momentary peek at what I would consider to have been her pure essence, and in that moment, I had a mother who was truly and completely capable of loving her little girl.

As I think of my mom now, especially in meditative moments, this is the mother I see; this is the mother I love. She was there all along, but just buried under "a big pile of shit," as she so delicately put it, as she came out of her essence and back into the tortured ego that defined her life this time around.

Thomas Merton describes beautifully this thing called essence. "Then it was as if I suddenly saw the secret beauty of their hearts, the depths of their hearts where neither sin nor desire can reach the core of their reality, the person that each one is in God's eyes. If only they could see themselves as they really are. If only we could see each other that way all the time, there would be no more need for war or hatred or cruelty or greed. I suppose the big problem would be that we would fall down and worship each other." [1]

Even with years of education, this forgiveness process took me 25 years. This is not easy. Understand that forgiveness can happen only when you have raged, grieved and worked things through sufficiently. This is something that simply can't happen before its time. But by including your unconditionally loving spirit in the process by means of lovingkindness meditation, your heart will be capable of complete forgiveness much sooner.

Jack Kornfield says, "Forgiveness means giving up all hope of a better past." It's true, isn't it? Being stuck in thoughts like "'it should have been this way," "he should have done that," "if only she had loved me more, then I would be happy," keeps us mired in the past with no hope of salvaging a present or a future. Letting go is a necessity; forgiveness is the key to letting go.

Buddhists believe in reincarnation, and that one's next life will be built on the karma earned in past lives. Reincarnation allows us to be reborn over and over until we become enlightened. Each life is filled with opportunities and challenges to learn the lessons that he or she needs to learn. In each incarnation, we have free will and can determine which lessons will be learned successfully and which will require future incarnations to master. In between lives, according to this belief, we get together with other souls to decide what roles we will play for one another the next time around. The concept of the "noble friend" teaches that the beings to whom we are closest will come back in relationships that challenge us through conflict to help us work on a given lesson. So all difficult people—the alcoholic mother, the cheating husband, the rebellious child, and the unreasonable boss, out of their love for us, chose to reincarnate with the express purpose of helping us to overcome our challenges. Now, how's that for a different way to think about the difficult people in your life? Whether you believe it or not, this certainly makes sending lovingkindness meditation much easier doesn't it?   According to the Dalai Lama, "One must exert one's best efforts not to harbor hatred towards the enemy, but rather use the encounter as an opportunity to enhance one's practice of patience and tolerance. In fact the enemy is the necessary condition for practicing patience."[2]

Whether you believe in reincarnation or not, having the ability to view troublesome individuals in this way changes the entire interaction. There is always something to be learned from looking at each encounter, especially those in which your buttons are being pushed. Our symptoms, mood states and interpersonal conflicts are filled with growth potential. So when I'm in the midst of a disagreement with my older daughter and she suggests that I should be grateful to her for not doing what she was asked, or for acting disrespectfully, I realize that, despite the fact that she is using my own philosophy against me, she is right. She is one of my greatest teachers.

Informal lovingkindness meditation has many of the same principles as the formal Buddhist tradition. Visualizing all people in your life, including yourself, your enemies and everyone in between and sending them (and yourself) love is the goal. This can be done any time, any place—sitting, waiting in line, pumping gas. You can send formal mantras or wishes, or use images of beams of beautiful white light. Or you can picture yourself hugging, comforting or taking care of this person. One of my favorite ways of doing this meditation is listening intently to music with loving lyrics, during which I mentally send whatever emotions arise to whomever the music brings to mind. I have made a few CDs that contain my favorite love songs specifically for this purpose. Music reminds me of everyone I have loved, and it gives me joy to remember them all and to send them my love and best wishes. This is a powerful practice that I recommend to you highly.

.   Informal Lovingkindness Meditation
CD # 2, Track #2
Music licensed through Megatrax Production Music

CHAPTER TEN

Tonglen Meditation

Tonglen meditation is one in which you consciously take on those things which you would normally push away and give away things you might hoard. When a friend, for example, is going through a difficult time, say an illness or a divorce, you consciously breathe this misfortune into yourself and breathe out healing, your love, best wishes or whatever your heart tells you will benefit this person. If, on the other hand, you are experiencing some happiness or good fortune, you breathe this out as a way of mentally sharing your happiness with others.

The practice of Tonglen is based on the truth that suffering is part of being human. Suffering is nobody's fault—not your mother's, your doctor's, your boyfriend's—it just is. You cannot avoid this certainty and running away will only make things worse. Tonglen is a practice of taking on and facing those difficulties—your own or those of others—fearlessly and with equanimity. This encourages the quality of compassion to permeate your life, which will not only benefit others, but will bring joy into your life and all your relationships. It is also a way to practice generosity of spirit. Your willingness to mentally share your own blessings will help to make generosity a more natural and satisfying part of your life.

Something I hear a lot working in the Emergency Room is, "Why me?" "Why did I have to break my ankle?" "Why am I the one to get pneumonia?" "Why did I have to get poison ivy on my face right before the prom?" And the bigger why me's, "Why did I have to get cancer?" "Why do I have to die?" Even people in their 90's come in saying, "I haven't been sick a day in my life, why is this happening to me now?" Regardless of our age and the challenges we face in this human existence, we don't want it to change and we don't want it to end. Woody Allen says, "Life is full of miserable-ness, loneliness, unhappiness and suffering and it is all over much too quickly."[1] Despite the realities that our lives show us again and again, we seem to feel that we are alone with our particular affliction, separated from the rest of humanity. When the truth is, it is our suffering that connects us.

Tonglen meditation is done with the understanding and acceptance that each and every one of us endures a certain amount of pain. The practice of taking painful situations into your self will make it more likely that you will be able to meet actual difficulties with peace and acceptance rather than self-pity. There is a great deal of energy in suffering, whether yours or somebody else's. This meditation uses this energy to open your heart.

Pema Chodron has written many books on Tonglen. She says that pushing pain away and grasping at pleasure are normal human tendencies. Either way, we are not being with what is, not accepting what is true, and therefore our lives are passing us by. Tonglen is a practice of going against our usual tendencies and doing the opposite. It is a practice of being exactly where you are at any given time and using that to foster generosity, compassion and peaceful acceptance of life just as it is.

As a practice of compassion, Tonglen asks you to picture someone who is having a difficult time. While holding this person in your heart, use the image of breathing in this person's pain as a dark hot smoke, mentally transform that suffering into a bright light of love and healing, and then breathe the healing light back to that person. Or, if you are having difficulties, breathe this in with the intention of taking on the suffering for everyone who is going through something similar. This helps you to move closer to pain rather than just enduring it. Pain has the ability to both awaken and soften you; compassion will naturally follow.

If things are going well for you, Tonglen is a practice of generosity in which you mentally send out your own good fortune and health to anyone with whom you want to share happiness. This can be as simple as sending out your joy of walking on the beach, having a good meal, or the peace you experience from meditation. What is important is your willingness to let go of your own blessings and shae them with others. Although this is only an exercise, mentally giving away your own good fortune makes it far more likely that you will do this in your life. Your willingness to share your own good fortune and love will bring you more of the same.

Tonglen helps us to accept ourselves and realities just as they are. Our silent, loving, right brain awareness helps us to realize that we have the strength to deal with anything. Helen Keller, despite her overwhelming challenges, demonstrates the incredible inner strength that we all have and the need to accept what comes our way. "Life is either a daring adventure or nothing. Security does not exist in nature, nor do the children of men as a whole experience it. Avoiding danger is no safer in the long run than exposure."[2]

The first line in the Simon and Garfunkle song, "The Sounds of Silence," is "Hello darkness my old friend." Like it or not, it is from the darkness in our lives that we learn our most valuable lessons and as such *is* our friend. In Buddhist tradition, learning the lessons is why we are here. Again, from Helen Keller, "Difficulties meet us at every turn. They are the accompaniment of life. Out of the pain grows the violets of patience and sweetness. The richness of human experience would lose something of rewarding joy if there were no limitations to overcome. Character cannot be developed in ease and quiet. Only through experience of trial and suffering can the soul be strengthened, ambition inspired and success achieved."[3]

In *Awakening the Buddhist Heart*, Lama Surya Das recalls a statement made by Chogyam Trumpa Rinpoche, "The more shit you encounter along the path, the better your spiritual flowers will grow— as long as you know how to use the shit as fertilizer." Surya Das refers to this as the "manure principle" and suggests that the best way to deal with the certainty of life's problems is to "bring it on... leap right into that sea of bullshit and swim."[4]

If you look around, you will see how much good actually comes from darkness, or those things that we consider "bad". This is true even in the animal world. The peacock is known to eat poisonous snakes, which despite making him terribly ill, will give him vibrantly colored feathers (and hence, all the girls).

Graham Greene, in his book *Third Man,* makes the point that tragedy often produces genius. "In Italy for thirty years under the Borgias, they had warfare, terror, murder and bloodshed; but they produced Michelangelo, Leonardo da Vinci and the Renaissance. In Switzerland, they have brotherly love, 500 years of democracy and peace; and what did they produce? The cuckoo clock."[5] Nothing against cuckoo clocks, per se, but heart wrenching tragedy and sorrow breaks our hearts wide open, propelling us into the most brilliant, loving, creative parts of ourselves.

When we run away from tragedy, we feel and learn nothing. By willingly taking on the pain and suffering that is there anyway, we remain in control. Again, Helen Keller says, "When one door of happiness closes, another opens; but often we look so long at the closed door, that we do not see the one which has been opened for us."[6]

Lovingkindness and Tonglen meditations open our hearts and help us to recognize and share the very best part of ourselves. With unconditional love as your meditative focus, you become more loving, compassionate and generous. Changing the quality of your life and the lives of those touched by your loving actions is truly the beginning of making this world a better place.

Tonglen Meditation
CD # 2, Track #3
Music licensed through Megatrax Production Music, Inc.

CHAPTER ELEVEN

A Meditative Approach to Nutrition and Exercise

A lot has been said about the food pyramid. Atkins, The Zone, South Beach and Weight Watchers are as well known to you as your name and address. All of these approaches have significant value, but they need not be discussed in detail here. The one thing missing in all of these approaches to nutrition and exercise is the use of the right brain's genius. The right brain helps you make the nutrition and exercise decisions, which are best for you as an individual. Our bodies are as different and unique as our personalities; there is no one size fits all. The information we need to make the best decisions for ourselves is right inside.

No book or health program in Mind-Body Medicine would be complete without including information on proper nutrition and exercise. As I contemplated teaching this as a part of my lecture series, it was with great trepidation, as I couldn't get past the following thought. "Why would anyone want to listen to this chubby, 50+-year-old junk food junkie, with sporadic exercise phobia talk about nutrition and exercise? Before I do this lecture, I will have to go back on that liquid diet again and lose 50 pounds" So, I meditated on this, and I realized that this thought actually formed the basis of this lecture because it explains why diets fail; and on *that* I am the expert. Not only have I personally always had a problem with weight, it has also become a significant national health problem.

The popular assumption is that people are overweight because of mindless consumption of huge quantities of food. The only truth in this statement is in the word "mindless." As discussed in Chapter 6, many of us have developed the unfortunate habit of mindless eating in which we shove quantities of quickly prepared food into our mouths as a response to stress, fatigue, or being too busy to nourish ourselves properly throughout the day. This food gets eaten with lightning speed, passes through our mouths, and is scarcely tasted, let alone enjoyed. Although this is a part of the problem, it is only a part of the story.

Beginning with "chubby," I will discuss each self-deprecating word in that statement and how it contributes to the problem. Not unlike many people who develop weight problems, mine was a less than auspicious beginning. I can still hear my mother speaking disdainfully that I was such a fat baby; I couldn't drag my significant mass off the floor to walk until I was nearly two years old. Although studies have shown that chubby babies often become chubby adults, there is more to it than that. The negative manner, in which these comments were made, made a huge impression on me. Despite being a thin to normal sized child, a significant part of my self-image involved being a fat person. When I look at pictures of myself as a child, teenager and young adult, it is inconceivable that this self-perception stuck, as I was a thin and attractive child. It is sad that I was never able to appreciate that reality, as this false, negative self-concept was all I knew.

I started dieting around the age of eight. When I was not on a diet, I felt guilty whenever I ate food. Assisted by a mother who reminded me of the fat baby story and her disdain for anyone with extra weight, I already knew the calorie count of every food and obsessively tried to keep my intake under 800 calories per day. Thankfully, it never dawned on me to make myself throw up; but the specter of fatness lurked around every corner, making for a less pleasant childhood and adolescence than it might have been.

As an adult, I have been amazed to discover how many girls grow up feeling this way. And yet, as we look back at pictures of ourselves in childhood, going to proms and other special occasions, we realize that there was no basis in reality for our perceptions. How sad that we couldn't appreciate ourselves just as we were, much of our youth being tainted by these erroneous self-concepts.

Despite overwhelming evidence to the contrary, one's fat self-image never goes away. I still remember looking in a mirror, dressed in a gorgeous wedding gown for my first marriage and thinking, "Why didn't I lose just 15 more pounds? Then the wedding would have been perfect." Sad, when what I should have been thinking about was why the marriage would last only four years. But that is another story. When I was in my 20's, I was 5-feet, 6-inches and weighed 130 pounds. Yet, I convinced a doctor to give me diet pills. I had no idea that Dexedrine, the diet pill of that era, was actually "speed" (an amphetamine). Lose weight, I did, and come to think of it, I was very productive. One can get a lot done when 3 hours of sleep is all that is required... or possible. An interesting experience, I don't recommend it.

So chubby is not only a body–image, it is a self–image, which can have a negative influence on one's entire life. This self image is life long, often despite evidence to the contrary. The thought of having a little extra weight is embarrassing at best, paralyzing at worst. The fact of the matter is that, in our society, people often don't take overweight people seriously; and even worse, overweight people don't take themselves seriously. We've all heard the comments indicating that overweight people are stupid, lazy, have no motivation and they're not valuable people. In fact, many people with extra weight, especially women, are embarrassed to seek medical attention knowing that getting on the scale will set the tone for the entire visit.

I don't mean to make light of what is a very serious medical situation. Obesity poses risks not only for a number of diseases but also for a person's quality of life. However, it is the unfair judgments that make most women feel that they can never be thin enough. Sadly, this usually begins in the pre-teen years leading to the devastating possibility of anorexia and bulimia.

This obsession with thinness is a relatively new phenomenon. The women whom Ruben painted during the romantic era, beautiful and voluptuous in their time, would be considered gross and obese by today's standards. The models today are unhealthily thin in appearance. Emulating them would be difficult if not impossible, not to mention unhealthy for young girls to achieve. Dr. Christiane Northrop points out that, in 1954, the average weight for Miss America contenders was 134 pounds and the average height was 5'6"; in 1982, it was 110; the average height was 5'11". Now, over 20 years later, the weight to height ratio is getting lower still. So, 50 years ago, the ideal fashion model weighed 8 percent less than the average American woman; 20 years ago, the model was 25 percent lighter, and that percentage is increasing still. Therefore, the body type considered ideal by our society's standards is unachievable for most women. Yet that doesn't stop many of us from abusing laxatives, diet pills, becoming anorexic or bulimic, or exercising to the point of completely shutting down their reproductive tracts. Dr. Northrop says, "The truth is, three billion women don't look like super models, only eight do; so… **What the heck are we doing to ourselves**??"[1]

It is not only size, but perception of size that influences the clothes you wear, the way you relate to people, and even your day–to–day emotional frame of mind. There is a cartoon showing a very skinny woman, with every rib showing, looking into the mirror and seeing a fat person. This is not the fantasy of some warped cartoonist; this is the reality of many women. Research has shown that people who have been overweight even for short periods in their lives will always see themselves that way even with concrete evidence to the contrary. Sadly, they literally can't see beyond the self-perception; how sad is that?

Chris Northrop discusses a survey published in *Psychology Today,* which found that 41 percent of women said they would give up five years of their life in order to be thin. Perhaps even more frightening, 80 percent of 10-year-old girls are now on diets.[2] This one comes as no surprise to me; I guess I was just ahead of my time.

The cultural obsession with weight contributes to a relentless cycle. Poor self-image caused by one's inability to measure up to model standards leads to emotional neediness, which in turn leads to food for comfort. Although food, especially of the junk variety, temporarily satisfies this need, guilt over having eaten it is not far behind. Weight gained by this behavior further feeds into poor self-image, and the cycle repeats itself repeatedly. The only place that the cycle can be effectively interrupted is at the self image step. Having a good self-image is one of the missing links in diet and exercise. The fact is until you can fully accept and love yourself exactly as you are, any attempts at making healthy lifestyle changes such as stopping smoking, drinking, and doing drugs, or beginning a healthy diet and exercise program are destined to fail. It won't work to approach these changes from the vantage point of self-loathing and neediness.

Ours is also a culture where aging is right up there with weight in terms of people's negative attitudes and misperceptions. Our culture values youth. Older people are not considered to be smart. Health is assumed to be on its way out. And practically everyone buys into the notion that elders have a decreased ability to be physically active. Although changes with aging are unavoidable to a degree, self-fulfilling prophesy will invariably lead to decreased physical activity, thus causing decrease in muscle mass and increase in body fat. The less we move, the less we are able to move. Some people, upon retirement, fall apart in no small measure due to the acceptance of these sorry cultural expectations, thus depriving them and the world of all that they still have to offer. It may take more effort to remain mentally active, physically fit and useful when the demands of career and children have passed; but there is no time or effort better spent.

Premature cognitive commitment, a term used by Deepak Chopra, describes the human tendency to accept the cultural expectation of decline as we age. Dr. Chopra believes that the aging process would slow down considerably if one could get rid of preconceived notions of what aging will do. A study done by Ellen Langer at Harvard illustrates this point. Ms. Langer took 100 people over 80 years old and sent them to a retreat in which they were immersed in 1950s culture for 10 days. They were given '50s styles to wear, food to eat, music, vehicles, and furniture—everything that would bring them back some 50 years in time. Langer tested each participant in strength, cognition, taste, hearing, vision, height and mood before and after the retreat. At the end of 10 days, without exception, every person was assessed to be five to 10 years younger in all categories, but returned to baseline after a few weeks at home.

Woody Allen says, "You can live to be 100 if you give up all the things that make you want to live to 100." This unfortunate belief is not uncommon and is patently untrue. Being told we shouldn't eat this, we shouldn't do that, especially as we get older, must be balanced with the crucial need to enjoy and have meaning in our lives. Happiest are those who stay involved in the outside world, find a way to give to others, remain physically and intellectually active, and have fun. Aging cannot be graceful or fulfilling with forced deprivation. Those who feel good about themselves and content with their lives make the best lifestyle decisions.

On many occasions, well-meaning adult children of elderly parents who come to the hospital ask me to reinforce the importance of strict diet regimens and limiting activities. They are not particularly happy with me when I tell them that enjoying life is every bit as important as a low cholesterol diet. Dietary and activity restriction, with the intent of prolonging life, means little to one whose overall quality of life is horrendous. Of course, making good dietary decisions is important and needs to be encouraged, but some reasonable compromise needs to be reached. The fact is when one is living a happy life, better health care decisions naturally follow.

My dad, in his 80's, still rides his bike 10 miles a day. Having had two bypass surgeries, three angioplasties, and bilateral knee replacements and taking multiple cardiac and pulmonary medications might give someone, less hardy, pause about such strenuous choices. But he chooses to live a full life; and good for him. My dad enjoys his life, making healthy diet and exercise choices easy. He is my retirement guru.

Having said this, it is also important to accept the inevitable changes of aging with grace. In Ram Dass' book on aging, *Still Here*, he likens going to the dermatologist for removal of old age spots to running outside with green paint and a brush to return the magnificent yellow, red and orange autumn foliage to its springtime green. Not only is this an exercise in futility, but it takes away from the beauty of what is natural. Though you may not consider age spots beautiful, there is great experience and wisdom beneath them. I for one have earned every wrinkle and don't plan to part with them.

It wasn't that long ago that sexuality in the elderly was assumed to be another loss that they would of necessity have to endure. The image of a dirty old man was great for a chuckle and nothing more. But in these modern times, folks have completely swung the pendulum in the opposite direction. With the advent of Viagra and now testosterone patches for women, having sex until the day you die and beyond is the expectation. Either way, people are not being given the chance to simply be with what is.

Ram Dass tells the story of a talking frog. An elderly man was walking down the street. Suddenly, he heard a little voice saying, "Kiss me, hey you, I'm down here, kiss me." The man looked down and saw that a little frog was making all this racket. The frog said, "If you kiss me, I will turn into a beautiful, voluptuous young woman who will make your every erotic, sexual fantasy come true." The old man considered this and then quietly placed the frog in his pocket. Out of desperation, the frog yelled, "Why won't you kiss me?" The man answered, "Because at this time of my life, I am actually far more interested in a talking frog."[3]

The point of this story is the importance of making peace with your authentic self. Although making the best possible health choices for oneself is much to be desired, understand this… that young, old, chubby, thin, happy, sad, you (the real you, irrespective of housing) is perfect just as you are.

Moving on to the next highlighted word, woman. Amazingly enough, despite obvious evidence to the contrary, women are still considered to be the weaker sex and inferior to men. Weight taboos are worse for women than for men. Men find overweight women unattractive and yet, for the most part, chubby guys still do all right for themselves. Dr. Northrop points out that assertiveness is a desirable quality in men, but women aren't assertive, "they're bitchy". A feeling of inferiority to men is one more thing that contributes to a poor self – image. Or is it the poor self -image leads to feelings of inferiority to men? Despite how this may sound, I am in no way criticizing men for doing this to us when we are so very skilled at doing it to ourselves. As Chris Northrop says, "It's a sad fact of life that women will never be equal to men…until we have large bald spots, pot bellies and still think we're good looking."[4] And you know what? Men have it right; good for them!

Food and emotions are intimately connected. At the end of a full workday, the woman usually makes dinner, taxis the kids from activity to activity, cleans house, does laundry, helps with homework, breaks up fights, and gets the children ready for bed. Facing this after a full day of work is a daunting prospect at best. With little or no time to take care of herself, fatigue and depression are likely consequences. When one is depressed, serotonin is low. Guess what temporarily raises serotonin levels: high sugar junk food. Other alternatives, including alcohol, smoking and of course Prozac, also provide temporary relief by blocking these feelings from our awareness. People who use food to fill the void experience a temporary boost in serotonin, thus making high-sugar junk food addictive. Unfortunately, exhausted females tend to be the unwitting addicts. The fleeting pleasure of junk food, much like alcohol and drugs, invariably leads to a junk food crash, causing guilt, depression and another craving for junk food.

Drs. Donald Klein and Michael Liebowitz, at the New York State Psychiatric Institute, have discovered that chocolate is addictive. (as if any woman needs a study to prove this one!) Phenyl ethylamine is a substance that is high both in chocolate and in people who are in love.[5] To me, this explains a lot. One might wonder whether phenyl ethylamine is also increased in lovingkindness meditation. This would not surprise me as meditation is also somewhat addictive but with neither the calories nor the guilt.

What is it that makes women so prone to guilt? Always thinking of the children, the spouse, and the parents, women often can't justify taking time to nurture themselves. Therefore my suggestion that the best thing that a woman can do for her health and well-being is to take time out everyday to meditate, relax or exercise is generally met with a look which screams, are you totally nuts? The day I picked up my first adopted child at the airport, one of the nurses in the ER told me that this day would be "the first day of a lifetime of guilt." My baby wasn't in my arms for more than a few hours before this warning became a reality. Never feeling good or smart enough to be the perfect mother, we worry and work ourselves to ridiculous extremes. Add to this a career and you end up feeling guilty for going to work and leaving the baby, and for compromising a hard-earned career by staying home. It's not unusual for a mother with a successful career to be asked what impact her career having on her children and spouse. Men are spared this kind of interrogation.

Fear of exercise is another factor that keeps a person from making commitments to her optimal health. Beginning an exercise program is an overwhelming prospect especially for people who perceive themselves as overweight. For some, going to the gym is embarrassing because they feel self-conscious wearing a bathing suit or exercise clothes. The "no pain, no gain" philosophy may also interfere with one's willingness to get started. So sad when something like yoga, which is gentle and good for you, allows you to start right where you are.

What about crash diets? One can lose a great deal of weight

quickly on liquid diets in which you take in only 800 calories a day. I have done this myself on a number of occasions, losing up to 60 pounds, only to gain it back, plus an additional 10 or 20 pounds within six months to a year of stopping the diet. Ninety-eight percent of people who lose excessive amounts of weight on crash diets tell the same story. Diets that require weekly EKG's and blood work to check electrolytes every two weeks are ill advised. This is not sustainable and is potentially dangerous. Weight loss programs and products are a multi billion dollar a year industry, putting it right up there with money spent on national defense. Studies have shown that only two percent of people who participate in crash diets will actually have a permanent change in their weight.

Most of us don't do well with deprivation, although this is what most of the fad diets require. Again, Dr. Northrop states, "It's a law of nature… for every diet there is an equal and opposite binge."[6] Deprivation has the paradoxical effect of making the person obsess about food more than usual, making the compulsive desire to stuff one's face irresistible. Alternating between depriving oneself and eating everything in sight, yo-yo dieting is ineffective and puts a great deal of stress on a person's body. It is also important to understand that with each drastic diet, one's body becomes more efficient at slowing down metabolism and increasing fat storage as a way of protecting itself from the ever-present threat of starvation with which it has become so familiar.

Therefore, with each diet, losing weight becomes more difficult. And yes, it is possible to gain weight while on a diet. I gained 10 pounds after putting myself on a two-month long diet of 10-grams of fat per day. And the last time I tried the 800 calorie per day liquid program, I went one month without losing an ounce. At this point, I have no doubt that I would be the last person alive during a famine.

If you answer yes to any of the following questions, Dr. Northrop suggests that you have what she calls a diet mentality.

- Do you continue to eat when full or eat when not hungry?
- Do you substitute caffeine or coffee for food?
- Have you justified eating six Twinkies now because you plan to start a diet tomorrow?

121

- Do you deny yourself food you really want or feel so guilty eating that you don't enjoy it?
- Do you starve yourself all day so you can have a big dinner at night?
- Have you weighed yourself several times a day, then feel depressed because you didn't lose weight in the last four hours?
- Have you committed the calorie and fat content of every food to memory?
- Have you ever taken diet pills, laxatives or diuretics just to lose weight?
- Have you begged your doctor for just one more thyroid test hoping to find a treatable, no effort required, and physiologic excuse for your weight?

If the answer to the preponderance of these questions is yes, then dieting as we have come to know it is not serving you and is making the situation worse. The only way to achieve optimal weight permanently is through slow and permanent changes in the way you eat and in your lifestyle. Eating a balanced diet, with no deprivation, exercising, and finding ways to fulfill yourself that don't involve six or seven cellophane wrapped goodies is the only way to do it.

Bob Schwartz did a study in which he put people who have never had a weight problem on weight loss diets to lose 10 pounds. As a result, these people became obsessed with food and gained back all the weight they had lost, plus and additional five pounds after the dieting period stopped.[7] So even being on one diet was a blow to these people's self-image. Imagine what multiple diets do to a person.

If, like most people, you tend to eat more when you stressed, you will gain more weight than when eating the same amount when not stressed. Remember, stress causes the production of cortisol, the stress chemical. In its attempt to ready your body for action, cortisol causes fluid retention and it stores body fat primarily around a person's mid section; thus, stress eating compounds the problem.

How does meditation fit into this? Beginning with mindful eating practice, there is no more satisfying way to eat than slowly, mindfully, chewing, tasting, and thoroughly enjoying everything that you put into your mouth. Even when you choose to eat chocolate or a bag of chips, do so consciously. Since you are going to eat it anyway, you might as well enjoy it; guilt serves no practical purpose. In a recent interview, Molly Katzen, author of *The Moosewood Cookbook*, says, "I believe that people who are overeating are not enjoying their food. I can't picture anyone getting too fat by eating slowly and savoring every bite. It doesn't matter what you're eating. It's how you're eating it that makes all the difference in the world. Opening up to the sensual approach will balance everything out."[8]

"Body awareness practice" is a term I use to describe a meditative silent witnessing of your hunger status, how different types of foods make you feel, and using this information to help you make the best choices for yourself. In this practice, stop and take a few mindful breaths, then focus on the level of hunger or satiety present. Using this information, eat only when hungry and stop when full. It's so simple, yet we go through much of our lives never paying attention or noticing what our actual hunger status is. Your inner being is smart; it will tell you which foods are good and which are bad for you, and will direct you to the best nutritional choices. The only goal here should be to eat for good health. Consider the possibility that weight loss can be a pleasant side effect of meditation rather than the frustrating goal that it has been.

Spend a few moments thinking of things that you enjoy doing which might be alternatives to mindless eating—walking with friends, listening to music, playing with your child, soaking your feet. Meditation can also be used with the added benefit of bringing you self-knowledge, self-love, and self-acceptance—prerequisites for taking the best possible care of yourself.

The more time you spend in the company of the real you, the more size becomes irrelevant. Don't let anyone suggest that losing weight is simply a matter of self-discipline. It is all about eating well, exercising and learning to love yourself. Meditation will help you to make peace both with your weight and with yourself. This will make everything easier.

Body Awareness/Body Image
CD 2, Track 4

Music licensed through Megatrax Production Music, Inc.

For much information about good nutrition, I recommend books by Andrew Weil, M.D. and books and audio programs by Dr. Christiane Northrop, the guru of women's holistic health.

A few well known diet plans are worth mentioning. The low-carb Atkins Diet can be effective for weight loss, especially in carbohydrate sensitive people. However, I have some reservations about its sustainability as well as the long-term effect of this much protein and fat to the exclusion of carbohydrates. In my mind, any diet that restricts fresh fruits and vegetables is suspect as the benefits of these foods have been demonstrated over and over again. Physiologically, the Zone Diet makes the most sense in that it recommends a balance of 40% carbohydrates, 30% protein and 30% fat, providing the ratio of nutrients which best addresses our nutritional requirements. The South Beach diet is a good compromise, severely limiting carbs initially, but gradually working up to a nicely balanced diet.

Eliminating carbohydrates all together is not a great idea but it is important to choose the right ones. Glycemic index is a measure of how quickly the ingestion of food raises blood sugar. Low glycemic index foods such as most vegetables, some fruits and grains raise blood sugar more slowly than do the high glycemic index foods, including all those with processed sugar, breads, pastas, and pastries. When blood sugar rapidly increases, there is a corresponding, rapid increase in insulin. Insulin causes glucose to turn to fat. Chocolate and other high-glycemic index foods also act like opioids in our bodies, causing them to be addictive.

Less insulin is needed for the absorption of low-glycemic index foods, making them healthier and less likely to cause weight gain. Fiber, also in the low-glycemic index carbohydrate group, is essential not only for preventing the discomfort of constipation, but for moving the cancer causing free radicals, byproducts of many processed foods, rapidly through the digestive track, minimizing their carcinogenic potential.

Dr. Weil repeatedly stresses that one must avoid partially

124

hydrogenated fat or trans-fatty acids, as these are the most likely culprits in free radical formation. The connection between trans-fats, free radicals and cancer and heart disease has become so clear, that there is beginning to be legislation prohibiting their use.

This warning aside, fats are an essential part of our diet, as they are needed for the synthesis of hormones and other vital functions. Unfortunately, the fat I'm talking about here cannot be found in French fries, sausages, fried chicken, donuts or butter. Our bodies need essential fatty acids, which can be found in flaxseed, canola and olive oils, green leafy vegetables, legumes, and citrus fruits. Omega 3 and 6 fatty acids are found in salmon and sardines. You may have noticed that despite having more low-fat food options available, people in this country are more overweight than ever, demonstrating, once again, that extreme diets of any description are bound to backfire.

Protein has a number of important functions. Many nutritionists recommend that a small amount of protein be included in every meal and snack as it not only helps to stabilize blood sugar, but it makes you feel satisfied longer. Small amounts of protein throughout the day are healthier than a big slab of meat at dinnertime. Although a small amount of animal protein is ok, if you are not opposed to eating it, vegetable protein is probably better for you. Protein is also necessary for the production of serotonin, dopamine and beta endorphins. As mentioned earlier, low serotonin levels cause depression while adequate serotonin helps keep us calm and focused. Dopamine, responsible for movement and emotional expression, is also enhanced by eating protein. Endorphins, the natural opioid substances that our bodies make in response to meditation, exercise and being in love, help to decrease pain and increase euphoria also require dietary protein for synthesis.

When it comes to making major life style improvements such as smoking cessation or changing unhealthy, stress-induced eating habits; your meditation practice is an invaluable resource. Just as the right brain is the best vantage point for silently witnessing your problems, it is also the best place from which to observe how much damage these unhealthy habits are doing to you. Taking the Ayervedic approach to smoking cessation as an example, Deepak Chopra suggests keeping cigarettes with you. Pay attention to those automatic cues, (like while drinking coffee) which make you want a cigarette and disassociate the act of smoking from the cues. Replace the cigarette with a healthier alternative. Later, if you really want a cigarette, have it, but smoke it mindfully and allow your silent witness to observe exactly how your body, particularly your lungs, reacts. After a while, full body awareness of the negative effects of smoking will result in an easier rejection of the practice.

This same method works for making better food choices. If you really want that hot fudge sundae, have it. But you must eat it mindfully, enjoy each and every bite, and pay close attention to how your body feels bite by bite. No guilt allowed. Feeling gratitude for the chance to enjoy such a tasty treat is a must. I guarantee that you will only be able to finish a small portion and at the same time, you won't be depriving yourself.

The benefits of exercise for your health and well-being cannot be overstated. There is nothing better for helping you to reach your optimal weight and physical status. Exercise speeds up your metabolism by decreasing fat and increasing muscle mass. Although exercise is also something that you do for its own sake, desirable side effects include prevention of cardiovascular disease, and increased energy and endorphin production. A decrease in pain, cancer, depression, and PMS symptoms will also be a likely result. People who exercise are physiologically younger, have better cognitive skills, a longer life expectancy, stronger bones and fewer fractures. Exercise makes your body more sensitive to insulin, thus less insulin is needed and you are less likely to become diabetic. Lower levels of insulin result in less fat production. And by increasing alpha waves in the brain, exercise helps you to achieve a deeper meditative state.

Exercise does not have to be painful to be good for you. It must be something you enjoy in a place you like to be if you have any hope of making it a part of your regular routine. It is very important not to sabotage yourself, as doing too much too soon serves only to punish your body and will guarantee that you won't continue. The only good exercise is the one that you will do.

Our bodies are designed to move and stretch. Healthy hearts, like any other muscle, need the exercise of pumping a little harder from time to time, and one's breathing capacity improves drastically as a result of a regular workout. A weight training program not only increases strength, but increases muscle mass, energy, coordination, bone mass and stability. Many people don't exercise because of fatigue, medical problems or pain. Although it may be counterintuitive, without exercise, you will actually feel more tired, have more pain and illness, and die sooner. But dying sooner isn't nearly as bad as the poor quality of life which results from deconditioning.

So, although it would be more likely for me to win the lottery and get struck by lightning on the same day than being mistaken for an aerobics instructor, my regular exercise/self nurturance routine consists of going to the beach, walking a mile or two, sitting and meditating for 45 minutes to an hour, 10 to 15 minutes of yoga stretching, then walking back. My life has been so much better as a result. But understand, this is not just another day at the beach. Walking briskly decreases stress hormones and increases endorphins. Meditation also decreases stress chemicals and elicits the relaxation response thereby protecting my body from the effects of stress for the rest of the day. Sunshine increases serotonin decreasing the likelihood that I will be depressed. Lovingkindness meditation probably increases phenyl ethylamine, the love hormone. Funny images often a welcome part of my meditation result in smiles and laughter, which also decreases stress hormones and increases endorphins. I often write and create my lectures during my beach routine; creativity and exhilaration are responsible for the manufacture of a substance similar to interferon, a potent anti-cancer drug. So this is definitely not just another day at the beach, **IT'S A BIOPHYSIOLOGIC ORGY!**

Like meditation, exercise is a commitment a person makes to him or herself. For those not ready to make the jump, you can always make your walking time more "productive" by listening to music or books on tape. There is no rule that you can't meditate while you are walking; I do it all the time. In fact, the Buddhists do a practice in which the meditative focus is each and every movement and sensation associated with slow, mindful walking. There is no better mindfulness meditation than walking along the beach and noticing the details of the sand, rocks, seaweed, water, sun, sky, and clouds. I have been doing this daily for several years and each day I discover something new and amazing.

Finally, yoga is meditation in motion. Don't be frightened by those pictures of people with legs wrapped around their necks while standing on one index finger. Yoga doesn't have to be painful or drastic. Prior physical conditioning is optional and age is no obstacle. Yoga is about breathing, quieting and centering. It is about being in your body and stretching. It requires focus and balance and asks that you gently push your body only as far as it can go. Like meditation, yoga is about being right here, right now and in my opinion is the perfect exercise… for everyone.

If you are thinking that you don't have time for any of this, all I can say is that where there is a will, there is a way. As with everything else, it comes down to a choice between living or just existing.

Self Acceptance
CD 2, Track 5
Music licensed through Megatrax Production Music, Inc.

CHAPTER TWELVE

Spirituality in Medicine

Whether one considers himself to be religious or spiritual or not, an interest in spiritual concepts and questions is universal. One doesn't need to belong to a religion or attend church to question the meaning of life or to wonder if this existence, as we know it, is really all there is. The universality of these questions and concerns makes one wonder whether the need for spirituality has actually been hardwired into the human psyche, and if so, why?

Sensing that there is some one or some unexplainable power or being that brings order to the universe comforts us from the start. As it turns out, those who continue to embrace a sense of the spiritual and engage in regular spiritual (not necessarily religious) practice will live happier and healthier lives in the here and now.

So, what is spirituality and why is it important? One universal spiritual belief is that we are more than our physical bodies. When one believes this, he is less likely to become mired in the day-to-day symptoms, pain and problems of this life. Taking this broader view, isolated difficulties seem inconsequential and of no ultimate threat to whom we really are. A spiritually inclined person entertains the possibility that that non-physical part of us does not die with the physical body. Whether you choose to call this part the soul, spirit or simply an energetic essence is irrelevant, as it is the sense that we are somehow infinite that comforts us.

That infinite part of us is the home of our inner wisdom. This soul, spirit or Buddha nature, if you will, is brilliant, all loving and tries in its own silent way to direct us in positive directions in our lives; but it can only do so if we are willing and we listen. Prayer, meditation, yoga, silent retreats, vision quests, and religious rituals are all ways of opening ourselves up to this intrinsic wisdom.

Spirituality also presumes a belief in a higher, unseen power that gives order and meaning to our lives. Whether one embraces the conventional image of God as an anthropomorphic being out there somehow directing us or the idea that there is some divine order to the cosmic universe, a person with spiritual beliefs is comforted by the knowledge that there is some deep purpose to our existence.

What has become known as "nonlocal mind" (a term adopted by Dr. Larry Dossey from the quantum physics term, that describes distant interactions between subatomic particles) [1] is also a belief accepted by most spiritual traditions. Non-local mind is the idea that our consciousness extends beyond our physical bodies and minds and has influence at a distance. What is prayer but the belief that heartfelt thoughts, wishes and emotions will be heard on some level beyond our comprehension, and have an effect on situations in our lives or on those for whom we pray? Some studies suggest that this may actually happen; but scientific proof or lack thereof doesn't stop us from asking for assistance in times of trouble, fear and sorrow. Even some non-believers say this is a universal human tendency.

Some people assume that religion and spirituality are one and the same. Therefore those who have become disenchanted with traditional religions often eliminate the spiritual aspect from their lives altogether. During those periods of my life when I have done this, there has been an indefinable emptiness which makes me yearn for that which truly gives meaning to this otherwise difficult and confusing human existence. It is usually in tragedy and sadness that one's spirit opens up, making its presence undeniable, only to be buried when things settle down. The most precious gift given to me by my friend Lynn was an irrepressible spiritual awakening, which truly allows me to live the fullest possible life. Yet, I belong to no organized religion.

Do you have a religious affiliation that helps you answer questions for yourself, which brings you peace, gives you comfort, and helps you to be the best, most loving person you can be? In your place of worship, do you feel close to something divine which fills you with all good things? If so, you are very lucky. This is a real treasure.

My German Lutheran family was concerned when, at the age of 13, I announced that I would be converting to Catholicism. Although an admittedly unusual move for a young teenager, the Catholic Church provided support and structure for my life that was not available in my family situation. The nuns and priests of my hometown parish nurtured, encouraged and helped me to realize my connection to something greater than the often painful details of my life. There was no place in the world where I felt happier, more peaceful, and blessed than when sitting quietly in church with no one but me and the sense of Divine presence all around me. I am forever grateful to Catholicism for guiding me safely through my teenage years.

As we enter young adulthood and gain the life experience that goes along with this passage, we often question our innocent childhood beliefs. Meeting kind, wonderful, loving people from different religious backgrounds, sexual orientations, or lifestyles, I had to question a religion which taught damnation for everyone who didn't believe as they did. As I entered adulthood, I found that there were aspects of my religion that no longer resonated with the person I had become. The very same religious rituals that I found so comforting years earlier felt rote and devoid of personal meaning.

Like so many of my generation, I became disconcerted with the shadow side of religion. I am not referring to the antics of individual troubled priests, about whom we have heard so much of late. I am referring instead to the deeply imbedded paradoxes that lie at the core of most organized religions. It no longer made sense to me that so many religions use guilt as a way of maintaining control over their parishioners, when in my mind, living a joyful, grateful existence, accepting oneself exactly as he/she is, is much more in keeping with everything that I feel to be Divine. Intolerance of those with different beliefs, characteristic of many organized religions, runs completely counter to the unity implied by the "love thy neighbor and pray for your enemies" philosophies they supposedly embrace. A truly loving spirituality, in my mind, should include the acceptance of all others rather than the exclusivity of, "believe as I do or suffer the eternal consequences." How many wars have been fought and how many people have been killed and tortured in the name of religion, when peace is what has been taught by all religious icons in history? Unconditional love is the very foundation of every religious philosophy, yet hatred is often what is practiced.

Buddhism attracts me for so many reasons, not the least of which is its tolerance of other ideologies and the belief that all beings and all their beliefs, however they may differ from one's own, must be honored. Thich Nhat Hanh says, "Every view is the wrong view if it is held as the only view." The Buddha never said that Buddhism was the only true religion in the world. In fact, he encouraged people to discover and embrace truth wherever they found it. The Dalai Lama teaches that each person should honor his/her own spiritual roots, as they are as important a part of a person as anything else is. He tells people to be good Christians or be good Jews, but to use meditation practice to become most authentically who you are. "Compassion is the key to Buddhism, if we can learn to act with compassion toward all living beings under all circumstances then we will undoubtedly be happy ourselves."[2]

In his book, *Wit and Wisdom of Jawaharlal Nehru,* the late prime minister of India said, "Let us think that the truth may not perhaps be entirely with us. Let us cooperate with others, let us, even when we do not appreciate what others say, respect their views, and their way of life."[3] Organized religions will be unable to bring us closer to God or to world peace, as it promises, without universal acceptance of this philosophy.

I am not advocating that everyone who reads this book become a religious dropout. In fact, if a religious tradition is important to you, "don't throw out the baby with the bathwater." My friend Barbara says to think of religion as a buffet; take what makes sense to you, leave behind what does not. The most important thing is that you make it real, make it yours, and make it personal, therefore making it truly spiritual.

If no religious tradition speaks to your heart, finding your own truth is a must for giving life meaning and for the peace that it can bring. Whether you meditate on the beach, attend church services, or pray, what matters is finding some way to connect to something greater than your daily existence. You will be happier, healthier and more fulfilled as a result.

My church is a beach near my home. This is where I feel the closest to what feels divine to me, where in the course of meditation I get answers to questions and comfort for concerns. I often bring my dog Rosie with me whom I call, only partially in jest, my "high priestess." No sacrilege intended. There is no better expression of unconditional love than a dog for his/her master. She is totally present, completely at peace, and exemplifies the Zen ideal of "beginner's

132

mind," as each and every moment is brand new for her. There is no carry over from the day before when she may have been fed late or left alone in the house for a little too long. In many ways, she is a better role model than most humans I know for the kinds of qualities which, if practiced half as well as she does, would make life much better, much happier and more fulfilled.

One's ability to espouse spiritual beliefs is entirely dependent on his/her ability to accept the mystery of what cannot be proven. Whether you believe that God is a guy in a white robe orchestrating everything in the beyond or is the ground of cosmic consciousness— the energy source from which all things come—or something inside each and everyone of us, we are required to accept without the ability to either see or prove; this is not easy to do in a materialistic society.

There are also the faith challenging questions such as, if God is all love, why is there evil in the world? Why are we here? Why do we suffer? Is there a grand plan or design? Do we survive physical death?

Teilhard de Chardin asked, "Are we physical beings having a spiritual experience, or are we spiritual beings having a physical experience?" How you respond to these questions determines how you will be affected by the ups and downs of your day-to-day existence. If you believe that we are only physical beings then symptoms, illness, and the disappointments, which are part and parcel of our human life, will of necessity loom large and have a far more devastating impact than they would for a person who believes that this human life is only a minute part of his spiritual journey. In this context, it is easier to accept life's challenges as the lessons necessary for the growth of the enduring non-physical part of our being. The impact that this belief has on one's sense of well-being is clear and the ramifications on physical health obvious.

As much as I have studied and practiced various religions, I don't know much. But I do know that Truth, with a capital "T" lies in what religions have in common, not what divides them—that at their core, all religions are pure love. The dark side of religion comes from unenlightened humans who have not yet recognized that core of love within themselves.

Recent terrorist events have made many westerners question Islamic beliefs. Yet, the Koran teaches, "Love for God is corroborated through love for neighbors, and in fact *all* beings, and that it is impossible for those who do evil to love God."[4] That the attack on September 11, 2001 was a truly evil act is clear. Therefore, it was not caused by the Islamic religion, nor did God cause it. Crazed individuals who misconstrued the whole point of their own religion to justify their own misguided and evil human agenda caused this horrible event. If you look at photo essays of that tragic time, you can see the hand of God in the walls of written condolences; the flowers that filled city blocks; the tears and compassionate embraces; the awesome bravery of the rescuers; the candlelight vigils; and the photographs of life going on, even as the burning and smoke continued in the background.

The fact that this was an evil act cannot be disputed. But it is not unlike the thousands of evil acts that have been and continue to be perpetrated by human beings now and throughout history. It's just that it took place here. We are blind to worldwide atrocities, especially those to which our own way of life has in some way contributed. We are all guilty of reinterpreting God to suit our own plans, ideologies and lifestyle. But the Truth is that evil will disappear when **everyone** gets the pure message of Jesus, Buddha, and the spiritual leaders of the myriad spiritual traditions... that **love and compassion are the point**. That spark of love, call it Holy Spirit, Buddha nature, Christ consciousness is within all of us. Evil will disappear only when we all recognize and live that **100%** of the time and not a moment sooner. I don't know about you, but I fall significantly short of this goal.

We all want world peace. But we need not look any further than ourselves in order to achieve this goal. Pointing fingers at the nation of Islam, the Nazis, or the Communists isn't as helpful as the deep understanding that peace begins and ends with each one of us. Love and compassion, the absolute requisites for world peace, need to be birthed person by person. This is the purpose of meditation, prayer, introspection and traditional religious practice. When we realize that we are all One, then and only then can we truly know this thing called God. The purpose of your life is to find that truth for yourself and live it. Living your truth brings peace. Inner peace brings healing and joy, first for yourself and then the world at large.

What do spiritual beliefs have to do with healing? Seemingly a

New Age concept, spirituality has been a part of healing in all of recorded history. The ancient Greeks got many prophetic, diagnostic and therapeutic insights in healing from the dream state. It was their belief that during waking hours, the ego is in charge, but while dreaming, the soul is active. They believed that the soul has more wisdom to contribute to healing than the intellect. Plato recognized that the emotional side of dreams was directly related to a person's health status. Aristotle agreed that dreams gave much information about bodily states. Dr. Galen actually performed surgical procedures based on what his soul told him through his dreams (a practice best abandoned!). Hippocrates, on the other hand, gave more credence to the intellect. He felt that disease had natural causes (not evil) and natural cures (not witchcraft); thus he is considered to be the father of modern (western) medicine.

In his book *Reinventing Medicine,* Dr. Larry Dossey explains how medicine changed from this to what we have today[5] He describes three eras of medicine that explain how and why medicine has changed throughout history. Era I medicine, or Western medicine as we know it, is the practice of curing the physical ills of the body using only physical means. As scientific researchers discovered surgical procedures and medications that had a clear, positive impact on disease process and life span, the concept that one's spiritual beliefs had anything to do with a person's health was dismissed as ridiculous folklore. By way of example, he tells the story of George Washington's death. George Washington died of strep throat, something practically unheard of today due to antibiotics. In attendance at his death-bed was a young doctor who said that he had just learned a new procedure called a tracheotomy, which would have saved the president's life. While praying, doing repeated bleedings, laxative purging and treatment with sips of sage tea, the president's doctor dismissed his suggestion as crazy, and the president died.

This was the beginning of many such discoveries that would prove, over time, to provide miraculous cures for the illnesses which plagued humankind. Life saving procedures, vaccines, antibiotics and medications worked so well that the effect that emotions, mind and spirit had on health and well-being were discarded as trivial, useless artifacts of an intellectually inferior time. Along with this came the expectation, still held today, that modern medicine could cure everything. The contributions of western medicine and research are undeniable. However, in typical 'throwing out the baby with the bathwater' fashion, the effects of the mind and spirit on the body are dismissed. As a result, Era I medicine is less healing than it could be by ignoring the vitally important non-physical aspects.

Francis Crick, winner of the Nobel Prize for the discovery of DNA, expresses Era I medical philosophy beautifully. "Your joys and your sorrows, your memories and your ambitions, your sense of personal identity and free will, are in fact no more than the behavior of a vast assembly of nerve cells and their associated molecules."[6] On one level, I can see the truth of this statement; but on a deeper level, this comment diminishes everything I know myself to be. It dismisses what I consider the most sacred part of myself. I feel that this is exactly what happens to us as patients of an Era I-western medical system.

Dr. Dossey goes on to describe Era II, or Mind-Body Medicine. Over the past several decades, we have rediscovered what the Shamans have understood for thousands of years—the impact that our minds have on our bodies. Shamanic practice is based on the knowledge that a person's beliefs and his physical state are intimately related and that by influencing the patient's beliefs by use of expectation and suggestion, his body will respond accordingly. Similarly, Anton Mesmer found that by making suggestions to a person's mind under hypnosis (a state in which the left brain is quiet and the right brain is active), disease or pain in the patient's body could be improved.

When soldiers returned home after World War II, many of them were physically ill. Western medical traditionalists at the time were at a loss to understand why so many soldiers returning from WWI were ill, when no physical etiologies were found. The term "shell shock" described the concept that it was the horror of their experiences in war that caused their physical illness. Emotions were in and of themselves capable of causing devastating physical distress.

The placebo effect provides the most convincing argument of the impact that our beliefs have on our physical well-being. Just the belief that a simple little sugar pill will have some effect is enough stimulus for our bodies to respond with healing. And yet even with all this, modern medicine still underestimates the importance of understanding and engaging the patient's feelings, thoughts and beliefs.

Era III, according to Dossey, combines western medicine, mind-body interactions and the impact of spiritual belief and practice on healing and curing—mind-body-spirit medicine. Ram Dass describes healing and the importance of the spiritual. "Healing is not the same as curing, after all; healing does not mean going back to the way things were before, but rather allowing what is now to move us closer to God."[7]

Era I medicine strives to make things the way they were, a worthy goal to be sure. But all-level healing occurs with the understanding that change, even in our physical bodies, is not without its purpose and can actually bring us closer to the deepest possible understanding of who we really are.

What evidence do we have that there actually is a soul or spirit present in each of us? Is there is some immeasurable, non-physical part of ourselves and what is it up to as we live our lives? Does this non-physical part survive the death of the physical body? If so, where does it go afterwards? Is there a God or some form of cosmic consciousness that orders our lives? If so how might it communicate with us? Of course, none of these things are measurable or provable, but in the rest of this book I will present material that certainly suggests that there is a lot more going on than will ever meet the eye. And that opening your mind to these possibilities may help you to view the world and your life in a more peaceful way.

A medicine that includes mind, body and spirit takes into account that consciousness is a more encompassing concept than mind or awareness. It re-embraces the ancient belief that consciousness not only acts on the body with which it is associated, but that it has the capability of acting on distant things and people (non-local mind). Hermes believed that consciousness is infinite and divine, with the ability to extend outside of the body. The Islamic physician/philosopher Avicenna, said, "The imagination of man can act not only on his own body but even on others and very distant bodies. It can fascinate and modify them, make them ill, or restore

137

them to health."[8] According to Stanislav Grof, "Modern consciousness research reveals that our psyches have no real or absolute boundaries; on the contrary, we are part of an infinite field of consciousness that encompasses all there is, beyond space-time and into realities we have yet to explore."[9]

Everyone, at one time or another, has experienced non-local phenomena. Have you ever had the experience of thinking of someone and they call you soon thereafter? Have you ever known something just from your intuition, or received information from dreams? Perhaps less common are well-documented experiences of telepathy, clairvoyance, precognition and prophetic dreams. Remote viewing, the psychic ability to find something or someone who has been lost, has been used successfully in many instances of sunken ships, buried treasure and even to locate kidnapped children. Such notions, viewed by some with skepticism, have been embraced by the most unlikely geniuses of our time. Albert Einstein admits that even his world changing, scientific discoveries came to him as flashes of right-brain intuition rather than hard earned intellectual pursuit. To quote him, "Imagination is more important than knowledge, knowledge is limited, and imagination encircles the world."

Stories of what are known as telesomatic events abound. We have all read or heard about people who have physical or emotional symptoms at exactly the same time as a distant loved one is dying or suffering in some way. Feeling faint, weak, weepy, or having a sense of foreboding have been reported, only to find out later that this was the exact time of the death or accident of a family member or friend. According to Mona Lisa Schultz, M.D., "Whether we call it a telesomatic event or empathy, an emotional umbilical cord exists between people and we pick up messages from one another. Some people are able to become more skilled at this than others and they call this ability medical intuition."[10]

Medical intuition is a fascinating phenomenon described in detail by Dr. Schultz, Carolyn Myss and Judith Orloff, M.D. Of particular interest is Carolyn Myss, who without any medical education is able to know from a distance a person's diagnosis being told nothing more than his/her name and age. Having worked several decades with Dr. Norm Shealy, she can diagnose with greater than

80% percent accuracy.

Although most doctors don't believe in non-local mind or psychic phenomena, they actually use it all the time. More often than not, physicians just know the diagnosis. Lab tests are often used to confirm that our intuition is dead on. Bernie Siegel says, "If you don't know the diagnosis one minute after a patient starts to tell the story, you're in trouble." This is why human physicians are so much better at diagnosis than computers. Although computers can store much more information, they, unlike human beings, are unable to pick up the intangible nuances and the subtle feelings that tell a far more accurate story than all the available lab tests or reams of information stored on a disc.

So, what do you think about psychic phenomena? Do psychics actually exist, or is this just a sleazy way to make a buck? I have come to believe that psychic phenomena are real; they do happen to us all the time even though we may not recognize them as such, and psychics do exist. The only thing that differentiates them from the rest of us is that they are more in tune with the energies and information that is all around us. The Jungian concept of the collective unconscious hypothesizes that everything that is known or has ever been known is out there in the cosmos and is available to anyone who has the sensitivity and skill to tap into it. A true psychic has the ability to tap into what is already there.

Let me tell you why I am certain beyond a shadow of a doubt that this is true. A few years ago, I attended a lecture given by Dr. Brian Weiss. He started by leading us through a psychometry exercise. Psychometry is the practice of holding something that belongs to someone whom you don't know and then observing the images that this object brings to your subconscious mind. Dr Weiss then guided us through a long, relaxation exercise (hypnotic induction) to bring the whole audience into right-brain awareness. He then asked that we observe the images that appeared in our minds, stimulated by nothing more than holding someone else's personal possession. I was holding the ring of the young woman seated next to me, about whom I knew nothing. Instantly, I saw quick and subtle images of a white or light gray Victorian house, on a beautiful street in what appeared to be a small, lovely city. I saw a little girl, about age seven, with black curly hair, playing hopscotch on the sidewalk with a grandfather figure looking on. I sensed a grandmother inside, although I never got an image of her face. I also sensed that the little girl's parents were both alive, but somehow not as involved with her upbringing as were the grandparents. As an aside, I also got a short but definite pain in my left mid clavicle (collar bone).

I was certain that the person sitting beside me would think I was crazy, but, I shared my experience her anyway. As I spoke, her cheeks flushed, and gentle tears streamed down her face. In fact, she did live in a white Victorian home in the lovely, small city of Northampton, Massachusetts with her grandparents. Her father was in and out of the State Hospital there for much of her childhood and her mother had to work all the time. Her grandfather would watch her play hopscotch on the sidewalk in front of the house while her grandmother, (whose ring I was holding) to whom she was very close, was always inside cooking and keeping house. She became very emotional because, in her mind, she felt that she had just been given a message from her now deceased grandparents whom she missed and loved very much. And the pain in my clavicle? This woman had fractured her left mid clavicle just six weeks before, and it was only now beginning to feel better.

When asked, about 75 percent of the audience had images that were very specific from nothing more than holding someone's personal possession. Needless to say, this got my attention. The details of my images were so specific, there was little doubt that I was indeed tapping into something, but what?

Several weeks later, in another conference, we were again guided through a psychometry experience. Believing that my first experience was nothing more than beginner's luck, I doubted that I would get any information from the watch that belonged to the young man who sat beside me. Again, feeling relaxed while in a hypnotic state, images flashed through my mind in subtle but rapid succession. This time I saw images of a split rail fence on a ranch somewhere out west. Beyond the fence, long grasses swayed in the gentle breeze and wild horses galloped. There were two women—one had long blond hair, blue eyes and was in her mid-20's; the other was in her 50's and had long gray hair. Both women were wearing jeans and cowboy hats.

So here I was in Boston, sitting next to a young man, having images of wild horses in the wild west, again thinking I must be crazy. After sharing my observations, I learned that the man's best friend, a 26-year-old blond-haired, blue-eyed woman and her gray haired 50-plus friend had just that morning left his apartment where they had stayed to celebrate Thanksgiving. They were bound for their home on a ranch in Wyoming where there is a large split rail fence beyond which wild horses run and graze from time to time. So does that make me a psychic or a psycho?? You decide.

Hopefully, by this point in the book, I have established myself as an intelligent, balanced woman with no evidence pointing to psychopathology. In fact, studies have been done which looked at people who have had paranormal experiences to determine if they are, as some believe, mentally imbalanced. To my relief, they were found to be above the norm in education and intelligence, although somewhat less religious than average. In fact, in standardized tests that measure psychological well-being, people with mystical experiences score at the top. As for my being psychic, in truth, I am no more psychic than the average person. What it points out, however, is that information is out there to be had. Level of consciousness seems to be the factor that determines how much one can pick up from what is apparently all around.

Ram Dass quips, "You just gotta get cable." In our usual ego bound state of consciousness we pick up only local programming, as it were; but in deeper states of consciousness, more subtle information comes through. Like cable or satellite hookups for our TV, the deeper our state of consciousness, the more channels we pick up. True psychics experience these states all the time, without any particular effort, giving them access to the psychic equivalent of HBO, Showtime or even STARZ! Ram Dass goes on further to say, "There's much more in any given moment than we usually perceive, and that we ourselves are much more than we usually perceive."[11] Edgar Mitchell, the astronaut best known for his walk on the moon, and a mystic in his own right, said, "There are no unnatural or supernatural phenomena, only very large gaps in our knowledge of what is natural...we should strive to fill these gaps of ignorance."

So what exactly is going on here? Is there some wild energy

blowing around us that we can tap into? Explaining perhaps Carl Jung's concept of the collective unconscious, the hologram theory hypothesizes that the cosmic universe is like a hologram. (A hologram is something, which, if it is broken into a million little pieces, each and every piece has all of the information that is in the whole). Just as each individual cell in our bodies carries all the genetic information from which the whole is made, the hologram theory suggests that each one of us, being one of the pieces of the universe, carries all of the information that is or ever was. The ability to retrieve this information depends on nothing more than the level of consciousness which interprets it.

The recent breaking of the genetic code offers further evidence of the feasibility of this theory. Everything that we know ourselves to be is carried on about 3 percent of our DNA. What is going on in the other 97 percent? Is it possible that every bit of knowledge of all time is actually stored in our DNA? A wild theory, thought provoking, to say the least.

If each of us is in fact a single bit of a greater holographic consciousness, then perhaps we actually do have access to the larger self from which we have sprung. Is this what is meant in the Bible passage which explains that man was made in the image of God? If so, then we may indeed have something of the Divine within. Deepening our level of consciousness, through meditation and prayer, connects us to the very source of love and wisdom. Now this is the kind of awareness that truly has the potential to change and bring peace to the world. Perhaps, as the sages have suggested, we are quite literally all One.

In a recent Gallup poll, it was found that two-thirds of polled Americans have had some sort of extrasensory experience; half report contact with the dead. Thirty percent have had visions; two thirds have had déjà vu, and one-third report having "seen" things at a distance.

The ancient Greeks believed that the non-local mind even extends to sleep and dreams, contributing creative insights and problem-solving ability. Studies show that ideas and emotions may actually flow back and forth between individuals while dreaming, indicating that we are connected to others even in sleep. Robert L. Van de Castle did a study in which he showed one person a picture with the instruction to send this image to another person while he slept. There were amazing similarities between the picture shown to the sender and the dream experienced by the dreamer.[12]

Most people have had the experience of knowing, without looking, when someone is staring at them. Described by many as a "skin crawling" sensation, William Braud obtained electro-dermal measurements of subjects during periods of being and not being stared at. The one staring was in a room in another building with the instruction that he stare at a video image of a person in a distant room during specified periods. Braud found that electrical skin measurements were significantly different in staring and non-staring periods. What this suggests is that one can change the physiology of a distant person non-locally, by merely looking at an image of that person.[13]

Synchronicity is a common example of non-locality. Carol Adrienne defines synchronicity as "an apparently chance encounter that nevertheless seems cosmically orchestrated."[14] In other words, it is more than a super coincidence. Have you noticed that sometimes answers to questions that you have come from a book that you just happen to pick up, or from something said on a radio or TV program that you randomly turned on? Have you ever had the experience of running into just the right person to help with something that you are working on? On a few occasions, I have literally had books fall off shelves with just the information I needed.

A friend who had just lost her brother in a fire described one stunning synchronicity to me. As she and her family were bringing his ashes out in his boat to be placed in the ocean, she took pictures of an amazing sunrise. At one point, her mother cried and said, "Oh my God, I got my dove!" Apparently, when her son died, she asked that a dove be sent to her as a sign that her son was all right. And right there, framed perfectly in a sunray-filled opening in the clouds was the most perfect dove shaped cloud formation, of which my friend has a picture.

To continue Ms. Adrienne's definition, a synchronicity is an event in which "forces come together providing just what is needed. It strikes the participant as special or unexplained by cause and effect and triggers awareness of divine purpose. The synchronous event provides external answers to internal psychic states."[15] My friend's mother without question got just what she needed, above and beyond what could be expected by cause and effect, without a doubt convincing her of some divine purpose. In this one moment she got the confirmation she needed, which continues to bring her peace to this day.

With an increased awareness of the existence of non-local mind and the deeper levels of consciousness that meditation practice provides, you will become more aware of the synchronicities and information which abound in the universe. Tuning quietly into yourself through prayer or meditation is the best way to sensitize yourself to help and guidance; perhaps this is how and where your prayers are answered.

Thomas Merton writes of a special type of synchronicity, which he calls spontaneous contemplative experience, defined as a moment of grace after which everything changes. I had one such experience some 30 years ago after the abrupt and unexpected breakup of my first marriage. After my husband of four years announced that he didn't want to be married any more, I became depressed. Though not suicidal, I had fantasies of being swallowed up by the earth, as if I never existed. Somehow these images gave me a perverse comfort. Although I remained functional in a manic, workaholic sort of way, the sadness of what felt like a personal failure was oppressive. Over-achieving perfectionist that I am, divorce was more than my self-image could bear. I spent many a night driving rather than futile attempts at sleep, or waking long before the sun rose.

On one such morning in early May, while sitting next to the campus pond at the university I was attending, my heart suddenly opened up and I was overcome with the overwhelming beauty of the cherry blossoms, now in full bloom. The heat of the newly risen sun warmed and brought life back to a heart, which had defensively shut down. Each dewdrop on the grass had its own sun blessed rainbow essence. Even the graceful dance of the dragonflies as they gently skimmed the water's surface and the swans floating serenely by filled me with a sense of wonder and joy, never before experienced.

This contemplative experience came unbidden just when I needed it most. There was a sense of divine intervention as these incredibly touching, beautiful moments helped me make peace with a devastating inner turmoil. This simple experience of opening was without a doubt that moment of grace after which everything changed, as from that moment on, I knew with certainty that I would not only get through this particular rough patch, but that my life would be wonderful. I will be forever grateful for that precious gift.

Who among us hasn't at some time or other asked God or the cosmic universe for a sign that would help give us direction or an answer to a troubling question? It is unusual, I think, to get something as dramatic as a dove, yet the signs that we ask for are generally quite theatrical, lightning bolts and such. We are often disappointed that we aren't receiving the answers to our questions in the manner in which we expect. Therefore, I suspect we often miss out on the truths that are right in front of our faces, amidst the simple things.

There is a frequently told story about an old man who was warned that he must evacuate his home in preparation for a predicted flood. The police came by and offered him transportation to a safe shelter, and he said, "I am staying here. God will take care of me." A while later, someone came by in a boat, imploring him to get out before it was too late. Again flush with faith in the Almighty, the man declined. Finally, now standing on the roof of his house, as the flood waters continued to rise, he was approached by a helicopter, offering him his last possible chance of escape. Refusing once again, the old man ultimately drowned. As he approached God after passing through the gates of Heaven, he angrily asked, "Where were you? I trusted that you would save me and now I'm dead!" To which God replied," I sent you a police car, a boat and a helicopter, what more do you want from me?"

A funny story, yet, we all do this. While searching far and wide for the answers that we seek, we neglect to look in the only place where they are likely to be found—within ourselves. God or the non-physical universe sends us messages, answers and clues all the time. But our answers don't always come in flashes of lightning or miraculously blossoming tulips in the dead of winter; they often come quietly, with little fanfare, in the most ordinary circumstances. Our lives, just as they are, are full of them.

In *Reinventing Medicine*, Larry Dossey reviews many of the studies which were presented at the Harvard University conference entitled, "Intercessory Prayer and Distant Healing Intention: Clinical and Laboratory Research, December 1997. The entire conference was devoted to research, which attempted to understand whether individuals could influence others at a distance, supporting the concept of non-locality.

The keynote speaker was Edgar Mitchell, former Apollo 14 astronaut and founder of the Institute of Noetic Sciences, whose interest in space travel was born out of his intrinsic sense of mysticism. Mitchell designed a simple study in which each day at a specific time, from his space ship orbiting the earth, he would write numbers, chosen at random from a book of random numbers with the intention of mentally sending what he was writing to "receivers" on Earth. They were instructed to write down whatever numbers came into their minds during this same time-period each day. Mitchell found there was a remarkable similarity between his and his receivers' number sequences, suggesting the possibility that information may be shared among individuals who have no direct contact and are distant from one another.[16]

One of the issues addressed in the conference was can people or things be influenced by our moods, emotions or thoughts? Bernard Grad of McGill University presented a series of experiments designed to address this question.

In the first study, researchers asked three people to hold containers of water, which would be used to water plants. Water sample 1 was held by someone with "a green thumb." Water sample 2 was held by a woman with depression (who actually perked up as a result of being included in the study) and the third water sample was held by a man diagnosed with psychotic depression. Plants watered with water sample 1 did the best; those watered by water sample 2 were intermediate, which did about as well as plants that were given untreated water. The plants given water sample 3 did poorly, suggesting the possibility that the mood states of the people holding the water were somehow transferred to the plants by means of the water. From this, the researchers postulated that emotions may influence healing both positively and negatively, even through an intermediary object, in this case water.[17]

In a second plant experiment, barley seeds were damaged with saline solution. Half of the plants were placed in saline, which had been held by a "healer" with the intention that the plants not be damaged. The other half of the seeds were soaked with untreated saline. All of the seeds soaked with untreated saline were unable to produce plants. But many of the seeds which had been in healer-treated saline sprouted and grew into healthy plants.[18]

In another study, mice were given a goiter-producing diet. Group 1 was the control group. Group 2 mice had a healer hold their boxes with healing intention 15 minutes, two times per day, six days a week. Group 3 had a little heat applied on the same schedule as Group 2. The thyroids of the healer-treated mice grew significantly slower than those of Group 1 or 3.[19] In a similar study, the treatment group had healer-held cotton wool placed in their cages and the controls had plain cotton wool. Once again, the mice with the healer-treated cotton wool produced goiters significantly more slowly than the controls.[20] Statistical analysis showed that there was less than one in a thousand that these results were due to chance.

In a fifth study, same size surgical incisions were made on mice. Group 1 had healer-held cages, Group 2 had temperature-adjusted cages, and Group 3 was moved about but with no healing intention. In 14 days, every mouse in the healer group had healed more rapidly than in either of the other groups, again with less than one in a thousand that this was due to chance.[21] One can assume, given that mice and plants were the subjects, that the placebo effect is not a confounding issue.

Humans aren't the only beings whose emotions seem to influence objects outside of themselves. In the Tycoscope experiments, baby chicks were imprinted to a robot. This robot's only programmed function was to move randomly through a room. The researchers put the robot-imprinted chicks behind a plexi-glass wall through which the robot could be seen. Unbelievable as it may seem, the robot now spent the vast majority of its time in the portion of the room closest to the chicks. They then put chicks who did not view the robot as "Mom" behind the plexi-glass and the robot resumed completely random motion.[22] Even without understanding the details of why this happened, there is compelling evidence that emotion, whether from man or beast, influences objects, animate and inanimate objects, to which they are somehow connected.

Many people believe in intercessory prayer, or prayer on behalf of another. Some studies have suggested that praying in this way may actually have some effect on the person for whom it is intended, even if that person doesn't know that he is being prayed for. In a landmark double blind study, Randolph Byrd, M.D., from San Francisco General Hospital, enrolled 393 patients who were told that they had a 50-percent chance of being prayed for by someone unknown to them. The pray-ers, chosen from several religious and secular traditions, were instructed to pray for a patient, knowing only his/her name and diagnosis, for one half hour each day. Results indicated that the recipients of prayer were five times less likely to need antibiotics and three times less likely to develop pulmonary edema; none required intubations versus 12 in the control group, and 13, as compared to 19 controls, died.[23] Herb Benson attempted a similar study more recently but was unable to reproduce these same results.

Elizabeth Targ, M.D. got similar results in a study of 47 advanced AIDS patients. The 20 patients who received distant healing intention through prayer had fewer AIDS-related illnesses, less severe illness, fewer doctor visits, fewer hospitalizations and improved moods.[24]

Sean O'Laoire, Catholic priest and psychologist, studied 406 depressed people and 90 praying volunteers. On 11 measures of mood, anxiety and depression, subjects who were prayed for improved on all measures. Also of interest was his observation that the people doing the praying improved even more dramatically than did those for whom they were praying.[25] This is in complete agreement with the studies on lovingkindness and compassion. A person's willingness to send loving intention to others will result in better health and mood for himself.

Qigong is the Chinese practice of cultivating vital life force energy or "Chi" (Qi) in oneself and others. By means of various movements performed with healing intention, the Qigong master claims to be able to unblock and create this energy in another, improving health in the person for whom this practice is done. This is also the theory on which acupuncturists base their work. Although there haven't yet been enough studies to convince the western medical establishment of efficacy, there is little doubt in the minds of people who receive these treatments that something is going on.

Researchers at the Mt. Sinai School of Medicine, who studied the Qigong practitioner's ability to influence biochemical reactions in muscle tissue, had an interesting observation. Standing five feet away from a Petri dish containing a few muscle fibers, the practitioners were able to consciously make muscle fibers contract 15 percent of the time. Statistically, the odds of this happening by chance are less than five percent.[26] Dr. Garret L. Yount at the Pacific Medical Center of San Francisco found that Qigong masters can also kill cancer cells at a distance.[27]

Though these studies are fascinating, based on their size and design I would not expect them to be embraced by the New England Journal of Medicine. And although it is not clear whether they actually prove anything or not, they do show interesting trends. Their main value, I think, is to show us that, even though we don't have enough data to prove the details, there is a lot going on that we can neither see nor prove. "Absence of proof does not necessarily mean proof of absence." (Rudolf Virchow)

I am not suggesting that prayer or intention could ever replace what western medicine does for our physical health and longevity. I am not planning to lobby insurance companies to pay for the services of pray-ers rather than for physician services, medications or surgeries. But I do feel that it is crucial to point out just how complex we and all beings are. Studies such as these suggest what most of us have always known—that we are more than the bodies in which we live. And that the "vast assembly of nerve cells and their associated molecules," of which Francis Crick speaks, is not who we are; but rather an elegant transducer allowing the physical manifestation of the essence of our true selves.

Taking the concept of non-locality to the next level, consider for a moment that if consciousness can actually somehow break free from its body and influence others, as some studies suggest, then one might surmise that it doesn't have to die with the physical body. This is one way to conceptualize the eternal nature of the spirit and by inference, life after death. Larry Dossey wrote, "Mind Body Spirit Medicine then cures the 'disease' which causes more suffering than any other, the fear of death."[28]

A recent Gallup poll indicates that 60 percent of people believe in an after-life, 30 percent of whom believe in reincarnation. A majority also believes that they have had messages from loved ones who have passed before them. After the death of loved ones, many people experience synchronous events that make them believe that their loved one is still around, albeit in some disembodied form. There are two possible explanations for this. The more concrete interpretation would be that our grief makes us look for meaning where there is none. A spiritual or mystical explanation of these phenomena, however, might be that after losing someone who is close to us, we are more vulnerable than usual, more right-brained, if you will, and we become more sensitive to what the non-physical universe is sending our way.

I experienced many synchronicities after the death of my friend Lynn. Decide for yourself which interpretation makes the most sense to you. Lynn and I had many conversations about what was happening to her and where she might be headed when this life ended. It seemed reasonable to me that we should decide, ahead of time, just how she would get back to me to let me know if all this life after death stuff had any validity. Being pragmatic, I suggested that she turn lights off and on from time to time to let me know she was around. Sylvia Browne says people on the other side will often do that kind of thing; who am I to argue? This idea was simply too pedestrian for the likes of Lynn, who said that she would do something much "sweeter" than that, if possible, to let me know she was there. She frustrated me sometimes; I wanted answers and closure, and she wanted sweet!

As we were planning her memorial service, Lynn requested that I play Eva Cassidy's rendition of "Fields of Gold" at the beginning of the service. When I asked what she would like played at the end, she said she didn't know, but that I would. I had no clue what she was talking about; I shook my head and continued writing her service.

Lynn passed away a few weeks later. A few days after she passed, I took my grief with me to the beach. I brought Eva Cassidy's *Songbird* CD and played Track 1, "Fields of Gold" over and over again, granting the oceans of tears, which had welled up inside of me, full expression. After the sixth time through, my CD player wouldn't go back to Track 1 and kept skipping to Track 5. Frustrated, I shut off the CD player, opened it and tried again. Track 5 again popped up. I had no idea what was on Track 5, but I decided to listen, and I was stunned by the following lyrics.

> *For you, there will be no crying, for you, the sun will be shining*
> *'Cause I feel that when I'm with you, it's all right.*
> *I know it's all right. And the songbirds keep singing like they know the score.*
> *And I love you, I love you, I love you like never before.*[29]

In that moment, I knew what song would be played at the end of Lynn's Memorial Service.

Lynn was certainly not a person who would tolerate too much crying, and from that moment on, I haven't felt the need to shed another tear. After the CD player experience, thinking that perhaps I had been given a message from the beyond, I carried on a silent conversation with my deceased friend. As you can see, I've come a long way, from left-brain doctor to talking to dead people! Be that as it may, I suggested to Lynn that it might be a nice gesture if she would arrange for a butterfly to land on my shoulder while I delivered her eulogy, so that I could 'spontaneously' insert a cocoon to a butterfly metaphor for a person's passage from this life to the next. Almost giddy from my own absurdity, I finished my walk, got into my car and headed home, feeling happy for a person who had just lost her best friend. Or had I?

About one mile from the beach, a yellow butterfly with a single black spot on each wing landed on my windshield wiper and fluttered at me during the five–mile drive back to my home. Pulling into the garage, getting out of the car, and placing my hand on the windshield, the butterfly crawled onto my hand and allowed me to carry it out to my back yard and set it free. Even while this was happening, I was *thinking*, nah, this just can't be; but I was certainly *feeling* something entirely different.

A few days later, while cleaning the winter refuse out of my pool, another butterfly, this time brown with a line of bright orange spots along its wings, landed on my leg, where it stayed some 20 minutes. I then walked into my house to ask my friend Jane if she noticed anything unusual. Looking down at my leg, the butterfly now resting on my upper thigh, Jane gasped, just having heard the first butterfly story. I thought it best to get a second opinion on the matter to be certain that this was truly happening and not just a figment of a creative, grief-stricken imagination. At that point, the butterfly flew off into my house, never to be seen again. As this happened, I became filled with Lynn's scent, with which I had become so familiar during the last several months of her life.

Amazed, yet still unconvinced, a few days later, I felt compelled to go out the front door of my house, where I found a tiger swallowtail butterfly circling around my front steps, practically banging into my front door with each revolution. As I moved into my front yard, the butterfly followed along and proceeded to circle around me again and again. I got down on one knee and placed my hand on the ground. The butterfly then landed and started moving ever so slowly toward me, flying away only when my dog, Daisy, came bounding forward hoping to pounce on this colorful little intruder. All three of these "coincidences" happened in the two-week period between Lynn's death and her memorial service. Oh, and did I mention that this happened in April in New England, earlier than butterfly season. Could this possibly be the "sweet" message that she promised? Lynn never did do the butterfly thing at the service as I had requested; such a display would be way too melodramatic for her.

Several months after Lynn's death, the night before I was to present my first lecture series, I was a total wreck. Before Lynn, I was completely and utterly phobic about public speaking. However, my fears had to take a back seat to Lynn's request that I deliver her eulogy. Furthermore, Lynn had also made it clear that it would be my job to do something to change medicine, impossible for someone who is literally tongue-tied when in front of an audience. So, the night before embarking on my public speaking career, I asked my beloved friend, "Okay, you got me into this, so, where are your damned butterflies now?" It didn't matter one whit to me that it was January in New England. The next day I went to Lynn's house to ask her husband for a picture of her that I could use in my presentation. Along with the picture he gave me a gift that "he had been waiting for just the right moment to give me," a medallion with, you guessed it, a butterfly on it. A few months later, that medallion disappeared. At first I was very upset as this tiny object was so meaningful to me; but then I was comforted by the thought that it would show up again at some time in the future when I really needed it. And sure enough, it did, just as I was doing my final proof-read on this book.

A few years into teaching my lecture series, after giving my spirituality lecture to a hospice agency, Julia, Lynn's hospice nurse, came over to tell me that Lynn had asked her what she thought happened after death. Being a Christian, Julia believed that she would be with Jesus. Lynn considered this but then said, "I think I will be a bird... no a butterfly, fluttering all around my friends." That is not something that she ever shared with me.

So, what's going on here? Is Lynn still floating around here in some other dimension that I can't see, but is still essentially in my life? As much as I would like to believe that, I can't know for sure. Or, is there some divine force trying to send me encouragement? Or, am I somehow drawing these things to myself through the power of my own non-local mind to help with the grief of losing my dear friend? I honestly don't think I am that powerful. I do not for one minute pretend that I know what is going on here. But I have become convinced that there *is something* going on and for me that has made all the difference.

The one time that a holistic approach is far superior to traditional medicine is at the end of life. Rodney Falk, a Harvard cardiologist, said, "Patients, regardless of mental status or irreversibility of disease, are treated until the bitter end when they lie bloated, bleeding and crushed after the final flurry of infusions and cardiac massage, death inevitably having caught up. In England, this peculiarly American approach to doing everything in life's final moments is viewed with incomprehension and horror."[30] Again, I must reiterate that this behavior is *not*, as it is often assumed, the decision that most doctors would make, left solely to their own consciences. We are often forced into this barbaric behavior by a society that demands it. This can only happen in a culture, which having lost track of the concept of the soul, rejects its own mortality. The futility of

153

avoiding the inevitable is responsible for a great deal of our suffering. The belief that we are nothing more than our physical bodies is one of the real tragedies of modern western culture and medicine.

A more holistic view embraces the notion that this body is the perfect and necessary housing for this part of our spirit's journey. Death and dying are as vital a part of a person's path as birth or anything in between. The primary tenet of mind-body-spirit thought, similar to Buddhist philosophy, is acceptance. True healing involves the ability to see that one is whole and that from the point of view of the spirit, life is perfect just as it is, including its end. Understanding that health and illness, pleasure and pain, light and shadow, and life and death are necessary and one's ability to embrace the dark side of life without judgment makes for the best lived life and the most peaceful death.

There comes a time in everyone's life when a peaceful letting go and a gradual entrance into what comes next are far more humane than the alternative of keeping the body alive, come what may. Death then becomes nothing more than the process in which the body is shed, allowing the spirit to move on to its next destination. Do you see how a person's life and death would be more peaceful with this belief?

A holistic approach to dying then, is one in which the person's basic needs and comfort level are the only medical goals. What the person requires most at this time is compassion, empathy and love. It is the best time for just being. There is no greater gift for someone nearing his life's end than to have the company of people who are able to provide a sacred, spacious environment of acceptance where the one preparing for his/her passing can complete any unfinished business then peacefully make his transition from here to whatever comes next. And there is no greater honor than to be the one chosen to give comfort and support during one of life's most intimate passages.

I learned so much from the wisdom and revelations that came to Lynn at the end of her life, but more than that, spending this time with her gave me the opportunity to connect with Spirit. This has changed the way that I view life and death and has reinforced the way I have chosen to practice medicine.

What is it like after death? Lynn often asked this question. I certainly didn't learn this in medical school; I don't even go to church

154

for heaven's sake. Yet she asked me anyway, fully expecting a cogent response. So, flying by the seat of my pants, I tried an interesting experiment, not surprisingly involving meditation. After helping her get into a relaxed state, I led her through a body scan. But unlike the usual body scan, I had her imagine that her body was being erased, gradually, part by part. When this was accomplished, I told her I didn't know for sure, but I suspected it might be something like this. At this point, all her symptoms vanished. She had the most serene smile on her face, and she fell into a deep and peaceful sleep.

The next day, while thinking about this exercise, I "just happened" to run across a passage written by Kathleen Dowling Singh. "Transformation in people who are nearing death is similar to what happens to people practicing contemplative disciplines and meditation. The time of dying effects a transformation from perceived tragedy to experienced grace. Dying offers the possibility of entering the radiance; the vastness of our Essential nature, meditation does the same thing."[31]

That is exactly what I saw on her face in that moment—a transformation from the perceived tragedy of this horrible illness to an actual experience of grace that shedding this imperfect body and moving on would bring. Because, you see, from your soul's perspective, death is perfectly safe.

No one knows for certain what death or the dying process is all about. But the reams of literature about near death experience and reincarnation provide compelling descriptions about what it might be, which is as close as we can get to glimpsing the unknown. Dr. Raymond Moody, Kenneth Ring, Dannion Brinkley and others have written spellbinding books on the near death experience. Some polls indicate that as of the date that Moody's book was written in 1976, 13 million or 5 percent of Americans have had a near death experience (NDE).[32] A NDE is what is experienced during the period of time in which a person's heart has stopped and for all intents and purposes he/she is clinically dead. According to Moody, the experiences of people who have gone through this are strikingly similar. Although there is no one element that everyone experiences, a few elements are almost universal. How far into the experience a person gets depends on how long he/she is in this lifeless state.

Most people, who have had a near death experience report an initial feeling of peace and quiet; a sense that the struggle is over. Next, many describe a kind of whooshing noise, which leads them into a dark tunnel. At this point, people will actually have the experience of leaving their bodies behind and observing everything that is going on in the resuscitation room, accident scene, or wherever they happen to be at the time of clinical death. They have reported in detail what happened while they were being resuscitated. Blind people can suddenly see. Others actually move to other parts of the hospital or to homes of loved ones. Once resuscitated, they are able to relay specific verifiable details about what was going on during the period of time that their hearts stopped. Observing the physical body from a distance, some have reported that they had an ethereal, light or spiritual body from which all observations are made. In this state, there is a sense of timelessness. There is communication, but it is non-verbal. And all reported that their minds were crystal clear.

Carolyn Myss tells an amazing story about a young woman who sustained clinical death while in a motor vehicle accident. She reports visiting cars, which were stopped in traffic behind the accident scene, while in this invisible light body state. She became saddened as she heard people complaining that this accident was inconveniencing them. Then, in the distance, she saw what was described as beautiful sparkling light coming right out of the top of a car in the distance as if it were going right up into the heavens. Upon visiting this car, she witnessed a young woman praying for her, which touched her very deeply. Soon after, she was propelled back into her now resuscitated body. As the story goes, the woman, in the midst of this near death experience, somehow registered the license plate number of the woman who was praying for her. When the woman was well, she was able to find the name and address of the praying driver, and paid her a visit to thank her for her kind prayers.[33]

The majority of people who have been through a near death experience also describe a beautiful white light at the end of the dark tunnel. Some describe this light as a non-physical being, God, Jesus, or other deity representing their own religious background; others describe this light to be pure love. People say this being or light communicates to them non-verbally is non-judgmental, accepting, loving, and stresses that the two most important things in life are love and caring for others, and acquiring knowledge. This light being then reportedly initiates a life review in which the person experiences a detailed, chronological, panoramic, emotionally charged review of his/her life showing vivid, three-dimensional, instantaneous images of everything that he/she ever did. The emotional quality of this experience is particularly striking as people can literally feel the impact their good and bad deeds have had on others. The saying, "my life passed before my eyes" is given a whole new meaning in this context.

Another frequently reported observation is something called the border or limit. There comes a time when a boundary appears, perhaps a body of water, a fence, or a curtain of fog behind which deceased loved ones are known to be. Most people get drawn back into their bodies before crossing over this boundary, having realized that it is not yet their time; but they all sense that there is something incredibly beautiful, loving and peaceful on the other side. The few that have actually crossed over are those who were clinically dead for a longer period of time, and, upon returning to their bodies, report peace, tranquility and reunions with deceased loved ones. No matter how far into the experience, all realize or are told that there are still things they must accomplish in this lifetime and are then rapidly pulled back into their physical bodies, often against their will.

In the thousands of written accounts of near death experiences, people are certain of its reality and importance in their lives. Many completely change the way they live out the remainder of their lives as a result. Having learned that love and compassion are the most important qualities that a person can have, people who have experienced near death generally become kinder, more generous, more moral and loving. They tend to become more reflective, taking the time to understand the ramifications of their actions on others. It becomes of utmost importance to do what is right, as this is what gives life meaning.   Mind and spirit are now seen as more important than the body, and seeking knowledge is paramount. Now more intuitive and empathic, those who have experienced near death invariably have an awareness of a life's purpose involving helping others. Equanimity is one of the true gifts of having gone through this experience.

A person who has experienced near death loses his/her fear of death. They are now convinced that there is indeed an afterlife and that the soul continues to develop, learn and love. Death is no longer viewed as the end, but is now seen as a miraculous transition to a higher level of consciousness, a spirit set free from the oppressive confines of the human body, like a cocoon to a butterfly.

The vast majority of people who have gone through a near death experience feel that what comes after this life is indescribably beautiful and filled with love. All agree, however, that suicide is not the way to get there. The heaven/hell, reward/punishment model of afterlife is generally dismissed, as 'bad' deeds of this lifetime are viewed as part of the soul's learning process. Much like the Buddhist philosophy of karma, the lessons of this lifetime present themselves again and again until one finally gets them right, not something for which we are punished for all eternity.

There are the nay-sayers, who explain the near death experience as nothing more than the physiologic experience of an oxygen-starved brain. But then how would you explain why people feel so profoundly different after their experience? Are we physiologically wired to be more loving, spiritual, generous, caring and peaceful after an anoxic brain episode? If so, maybe the only way to achieve world peace is to deprive the world of oxygen for 15 or 20 minutes and see what happens!

August L. Reader, M.D., a NDE survivor said, "I have explored many of these paths, from Kaballism to Buddhism, from Shamanism to yoga… the final common path is the same. In the end, we each have to face the moment of transition to the next plane of existence. The more we know of it, the easier it is to cope with the everyday stresses of life. In that is healing—spiritually, psychologically and physically for the individual. For once you learn how to die you may then be able to fully live."[34]

In my lectures, I keep hoping that someone will ask the question; what if none of this stuff is true, what if there is no soul, what if the death of this human body really is the end? My answer would be, wouldn't that be all the more reason to live life as if it were? For if we truly have only one shot at life, why would we not want to live it in the best way we possibly can? Taking what comes in stride, learning what we can from our problems rather than running away or fighting them promises the best quality of life possible in the here and now. Regardless of what you believe, living a life that is filled with love and enriched by spiritual principles and attitudes is a win-win situation. But the fact is, it's all a mystery…it's supposed to be. So as with everything else, how you choose to interpret and live your life all comes back to personal choice.

No one can say for sure whether the near death experience is what happens during actual death, as those experiencing the latter don't come back and tell their stories, to the best that our limited brains can discern. But the lessons learned from them are profound nonetheless. It is clear that a life devoted to love, kindness, generosity, compassion, knowledge and gratitude promises the best possible life right here and right now, making the concept of afterlife an optional, though very rich icing on the cake.

Life Review Meditation
CD #2, Track #6
Music licensed through Megatrax Production Music, Inc.

The controversial topic of reincarnation provides another philosophy about the ongoing nature of the human spirit. Reincarnation was actually a part of Christian doctrine until the fourth century, when church and government leaders felt that if the parishioners thought they could take human birth over and over again, they would be less obedient. Fearing that disobedience was a threat to the stability of the empire, Emperor Constantine, a politician, eradicated reincarnation from Christian doctrine. Two hundred years later, the Second Council of Constantinople officially declared reincarnation heresy.

Judaism followed suit, dropping reincarnation in the early 1800's, as they wished to be accepted by western society; although the Orthodox and Chasidic communities embrace this belief to this day. Rabbi Moshe Chaim Luzzatto, accepted as the father of modern Hebrew literature, was persecuted for his belief that, "A single soul can be reincarnated a number of times in different bodies, in this manner, it can rectify the damage done in previous incarnations. Similarly, it can also attain perfection that was not attained in its previous incarnations."

This is in total agreement with the Buddhist and Hindu concept of karma, which states that there is no heaven or hell. Instead, each incarnation provides the opportunity to correct mistakes of the past all for the purpose of obtaining enlightenment. Most people who have had a near death experience, irrespective of their religious background, also have this belief.

It is ironic that the differences in religious beliefs responsible for so much hatred and violence in the world were nearly identical so many centuries ago. Every religion professes love and compassion as its foundation. So what is all the fighting about anyway? The teachings of Buddha and Jesus are amazingly similar in ideology.

Of late, through the work of Brian Weiss, M.D., Ian Stevenson and others, there has been a resurgence of interest in the topic as modern day "evidence" of reincarnation has surfaced. Dr. Weiss' entrée into this field is a fascinating story unto itself, described in detail in his first book, *Many Lives, Many Masters.*[35] A basic scientist, Dr. Weiss started his career as a physicist, not at all the kind of person who would be attracted to this particular field of interest. Following medical school and residency in psychiatry, Dr. Weiss began a traditional psychiatric practice; that is until he met Catherine. Catherine was a particularly challenging patient. Paralyzed by dozens of phobias, Catherine was scarcely able to function in the world. Not making any progress with traditional psychotherapy, Dr. Weiss tried hypnosis, hoping to uncover repressed early childhood traumas thought responsible for her devastating state. During one such session, Dr. Weiss asked Catherine, "When was the first time that this phobia became a problem for you?" She then went into specific detail about events that clearly took place a few hundred years ago, at which point Weiss initially dismissed her ramblings as being that of a seriously disturbed person. But something caught his attention. The phobia that Catherine had been working on had vanished. When asked the same question, week after week, Catherine would relay inciting incidents from past times, all in magnificent detail. And week after week, she would free herself from one disabling phobia after another.

Still not certain what was going on here, Weiss continued what, for Catherine had, become a very effective therapy. In one session, Catherine described what appeared to be a memory of an in-between life state. In this "memory", she spoke of the "masters", spirit guides of sorts who explained to her many of the mysteries of life. In this state, she was also able to tell Dr. Weiss many details of his own life that would not be available to her by ordinary means. That was when Weiss knew beyond a shadow of a doubt that his own life and psychiatric practice would take a very different direction.

What has become known as past life regression therapy has become a major part of Dr. Weiss' psychiatric practice. He has written several books about his experience and observations working with hundreds of patients who, when hypnotized, have amazing often historically verifiable memories. In his private practice, about 40 percent of patients will recall their past lives when hypnotized while the remaining 60 percent will be brought back to earlier times of their current life.

One intriguing aspect of this approach to therapy is that when past life memories come up, symptom improvement is almost instantaneous and dramatic. Phobias, stress-related conditions, ulcers, musculoskeletal pain, headaches, arthritis, allergies and asthma are only a few of the conditions, which can apparently be treated successfully by this type of therapy.

Does the fact that some people get better after this therapy prove the existence of reincarnation? Maybe, maybe not. At the very least, this method seems to uncover important psychological information, otherwise inaccessible. Once the feelings (memories) are out, in whatever form, they can now be addressed. Perhaps putting it in a past life context gets important psycho-emotional material out in a less threatening way than uncovering traumas which are too close for comfort. But what is interesting is that a person doesn't need to believe in reincarnation to have beneficial effect from the process.

Having had the opportunity to study with Dr. Weiss, I can tell you that this is truly a fascinating experience. Using deep relaxation techniques, he directs his students back to infancy and childhood, using suggestion to bring the person into times one, two, three hundred years ago. Indeed, you do see yourself in much the same subtle manner that I described in my psychometry exercises, in a different time, different body and in different relationships. Often, you can even recognize people who are in your current life, in different relationships with you in past lives.

You may be asking yourself are these actual past lives or just imagination? Or, as hologram theory suggests, are we privy in some inexplicable way to everything that everyone has known or experienced since time began? Was Carl Jung onto something when he proposed his theory of the collective unconscious? Who knows? But, ponder the following historically verifiable examples from Dr. Weiss' book, *Many Lives, Many Masters.*

Jenny was age 26 when she started having images of a life in Ireland some 60-70 years ago. So vivid and specific were the details of her memories that she decided to go to Ireland and find the spot and the people that she had so clearly remembered. She easily found the town, street and very home in which she lived several decades previously. She knocked on the door where three now elderly people whose names she knew as well as her own greeted her; they were in fact, her children from her last lifetime. Whoa, could this really be possible?

How about this? A couple living in New York had two-year-old twins, who seemed to be speaking an actual foreign language to one another. The parents had never heard a language that sounded anything like this one. Perplexed, they brought the twins to be evaluated by language a specialist. Come to find out, the twins were speaking fluent Aramaic, the language spoken at the time of Jesus.

Dr. Weiss and Ian Stevenson describe children who have skills they couldn't possibly have with their current life experience. How can you explain a three-year-old boy with knowledge about how to fly and repair a World War II airplane? Or a little girl who knows how to assemble rifles? There are volumes written about what children know and remember, yet who can explain it, for sure? Reincarnation provides one plausible explanation.

The Dalai Lama was recognized at the age of two as the reincarnation of the previous Dalai Lama. The recognition of tulkus, or reincarnated Buddhist leaders, is a complex process, requiring many complicated steps and rigorous tests. But when complete, there is little doubt in the minds of the Buddhist people that their beloved past teacher has returned to them in a new form.

As amazing as past life images are, for me, the information gleaned from people's memories of the between-life state are the most compelling, as they provide the most insight into the existential questions of the meaning of life—why we are here and how we can best live our lives.

Dr. Weiss' book *Messages from the Masters* explains what he and his patients have learned. According to the "Masters," (beings encountered while in the in between life state) we choose those souls who will be our parents, friends and adversaries in our next life. We travel in what they call soul groups, reincarnating again and again with the same group of people, although the relationships change from lifetime to lifetime. In other words, the person who is your best friend in this life may have been your sister, mother, or neighbor in a previous incarnation. According to the Masters, when you meet someone with whom you have an instant connection, be it positive or negative, this is due to soul recognition.

Remember the Buddhist teaching of the noble friend? The "Masters" say that those people who are the most difficult to deal with and who cause us the most pain are souls to whom we are closest. They play these challenging roles with the sole purpose of teaching us the lessons that our souls need to learn for our own ultimate enlightenment.

The life review is the beginning of the process of figuring out what you have mastered and what still needs work. What Carolyn Myss refers to as "sacred contracts," your next incarnation is planned to provide opportunities to master every single lesson that your soul needs to learn. Every detail of each and every one of our lives has purpose to this end.

One argument against reincarnation is that religious scriptures tell us that we have free will. So, where does free will come in if our lives are already planned? It's right here. As we are presented with the plethora of life's challenges, we can choose to learn, or we can choose the easy way out and put it off for more subsequent lifetimes; either way, there is free will and the choice is always our own.

Lynn's Legacy

The teachings of the Masters, congruent with the knowledge gained from near death experiences, form the basis of the spiritual part of a mind-body-spirit approach to medicine. For if one can understand and accept that life is endless and we never die, we just pass through different phases and levels of consciousness. And if we accept that we as human beings have many dimensions and that God or the Divine however you define it, is within each and every one of us, then we will truly be able to accept what is with grace.

So, how does all this tie together? Biophysiology of stress and emotion, mindfulness, imagery, lovingkindness, near death experience, reincarnation, and spirituality are all ways to get closer to knowing the real you—the God-like, brilliant, loving part of yourself. These are all approaches that help you to look inside yourself and see deeply; greater wisdom, joy and peace cannot help but follow.

The writings in this book and the CD meditations have been created with the express purpose of reminding you of something that you have always known but may have lost sight of in the course of this challenging human experience, and; that is how much meaning there is in this life. Everything we do and everything that happens to us, including our relationships, friendships, joys, sorrows, and even tragedies, are in our lives for the purpose of enhancing our spiritual growth. If you can wrap your brain around the concept that every detail of your life is there for your soul's growth and enlightenment, then you will be less likely to feel stressed, depressed, or unhappy. If challenges and death itself are nothing more than transitions into higher states of consciousness, then the most challenging of life experiences, instead of throwing us into a depressive tailspin, can be viewed as a time of enormous personal growth and new beginnings.

No matter how much scientific research is done, some things cannot be proven—the existence of the soul, life after death, reincarnation, is there a God. Do we burn in Hell forever for having committed bad deeds? Will those of us who are deemed worthy live in Heaven for all eternity? These are things that can never be known for sure; at least while we are all limited humans stumbling around on the earth plane, and that is how it is supposed to be. But acceptance of the mysteries even without scientific proof brings with it an inner peace, which is simply not possible otherwise. This is grace.

Spirituality in Medicine

Madeline L'Engle wrote, "I do not want ever to be indifferent to the joys and beauties of this life. For through these, as through pain, we are enabled to see purpose in randomness, pattern in chaos. We do not have to understand in order to believe that behind the mystery and fascination there is love."

What is important is that you discover your own truths, whether through meditation, prayer, yoga, hypnosis, past life regression therapy, your own religious tradition or even a near death experience. Your own truth is your God-given gift; your job is simply to live it and give it to the world.

My sense of the real cause of stress-induced illness/symptoms is that we must live a life which is congruent with what our inner being (or soul) is trying to tell us. Discrepancy between the actions of the personality and the wishes of the non-physical spirit is what causes us to suffer. Meditation, or any of the methods described in this book, acquaints us with our spirits, maybe for the very first time. Balance and healing can only occur when our personality and spirit are in sync; it is that simple.

What is your life's purpose? To answer this question, you must recognize the need for personality/spirit congruency. When you do, the more you get to know the real you, the more apparent your life's purpose becomes; it's quite easy really… Pay attention to your heart: it talks incessantly when you are alone in silence. Do what you love. One cannot accomplish a purpose without a passion. And finally, give the world the benefit of what you love… out of love for the world. There are only a few things that I know for certain, but this is one… *anything* done from a place of total love cannot fail.

Mahatma Gandhi said, "My life is my message." This is true for everyone. Your life is your message; your life is your spiritual practice. Everything that you know and everything that you are is your gift to give to the world. This is your purpose; this is the path to true happiness; this is the real thing.

One doesn't have to be Gandhi or a Mother Teresa to make a difference in the world; it can be as simple as this. *Miss Rumphius*[36], the main character in Barbara Cooney's wonderful children's book, was told by her grandfather that there were three things that she must do in her life. First, she must travel to faraway places; second, live by the sea; and third, do something to make the world a more beautiful place. After traveling to many exotic places, Miss Rumphius settled in a tiny cottage by the sea. As she grew older and more infirm, she looked out her window at some lovely lupines growing beneath her window and realized that she hadn't yet done what was the most important of her grandfather's instructions. Inspired by the flowers, she sent away for bags and bags of lupine seeds and spent her remaining days broadcasting seeds for miles around. Every spring, there was an ever expanding lush carpet of color representing one woman's love for the world.

Miss Rumphius was a gift to my daughter from my friend Beth, who died from stomach cancer 10 years before Lynn. In many ways, Lynn was the real life Miss Rumphius. Everyone appreciated her acres of beautiful flowers. Having harvested the seeds from her last garden to give to friends and loved ones at her memorial service, there are now hundreds of gardens that continue to be graced with memories of Lynn. But flowers weren't the only seeds planted by this incredible woman. She also planted the seeds of her vision to improve medicine; and as such, this book is her legacy.

In writing this book, I have come to realize that this is also my mother Claire's legacy, for if I can teach what she never understood, that true health and happiness can never come from other people or externals, both of our lives will have been worthwhile. It is all about personal responsibility and understanding that, when all is said and done, the quality of our lives depends on how we *choose* to perceive our reality, and that we must make conscious decisions to develop the loving, caring, positive attitudes that make our lives worthwhile, no matter what is going on around us. Goethe said, "Our friends show us what we can do, our enemies show us what we must do." This is something that I must teach.

People at the end of their lives, no longer needing success, material goods, fame, fortune, power or any of the stuff of life, have such pure perspective on what is important; therefore, death bed wisdom gets as close to one's soul as a person can get in this lifetime. In our last meditative exercise, I asked Lynn to enter this experience fully so that I could share what she learned on her journey with her friends and loved ones at her memorial service. I know she would be honored to have her words gently guide you into the last meditation of this book.

Lynn told me that, believe it or not, there were actually some good things about the process of facing her death. Her journey had been hard fought, but she wanted to share some of the truths that she discovered as her final gift, in the hope that they might in some small measure make others' lives easier. First she wanted us to understand that as human beings, we somehow think that we are our physical bodies, that it is the physical, which makes us invincible, when in fact our invincibility is deep inside where no one else can see. She wants us to open ourselves up to all the love that is out there for us and not be afraid of asking for help. She asks you to believe in your inner voice and allow it to guide you through your life. Strive for the truth, which is always less frightening than the unknown. Realize that everything you need is right there within you. All you have to do is look and you will find it; it is closer than you can possibly imagine. Don't ever let a disease become who you are, only something you have to deal with and learn from. Work hard to control anger but never settle for what's clearly inequitable – you deserve better than that. Find happiness in simple things.

The process of being sick and dying not only made Lynn think more deeply about her relationships with her family and friends, but she came to understand that, though her physical body would stop functioning, her spirit would go on. In the end, she knew that it was just her time to move on. Despite never having embraced any particular religious belief, she believed that she was going to a beautiful place full of light and love—a place where she would experience perfect health of mind and spirit.

All of us, still entrenched in our human existence, would see the terminal illness of a 40-year-old mother and friend as a tragedy and gross injustice. Lynn, however, understood the difference between human and divine justice. Over the many months of her illness, she came to accept the divine; she aligned with her soul.

Lynn asked me to tell everyone that she loved that she was certain that we would all be with her again and that she will be there to meet us when it is our time to move on. That in the context of an eternity, we will be with her in a very short time – the blink of an eye.

But until that time, she has no doubt that she will be with us in spirit and continue to be a warm, loving part of each and every one of our lives.

She has kept her promise, as I have never been closer to her.

Final Summary Meditation
CD #2, Track 7
Music licensed through Megatrax Production Music, Inc.

Endnotes

Chapter 2

1. Richard J. Davidson., et al, "Alterations in Brain and Immune Function Produced by Mindfulness Meditation," *Journal of Psychosomatic Medicine,* (2003): 65:564-570.

Chapter 3

1. J. K. Kiecolt-Glaser, et al, "Marital Quality, marital disruption and immune function*,*" *Psychosomatic Medicine*, 1987: 49:13-34.
2. J. K. Kiecolt-Glaser, et al, "Modulation of Cellular Immunity in medical students," *Journal of Behavioral Medicine*, February (1986): 9(1).
3. S. Zheng, et al, "The stress reaction induced by intensive noise exposure in rats," *Spac Med Med Eng* (Beijing), 10 October (1997), (5): 333-6.
4. S. C. Kobasa, "Stressful life events: personality and health. An inquiry into hardiness," *Journal of Personality and Social Psychology* 1979b, 37: 1-11.
5. L. S. Berk, et al, "Neuroendocrine and Stress Hormone Changes During Mirthful Laughter," *American Journal of Medical Science* December (1989), 298 (5): 390-6.
6. P. Ekman, and R. J. Davidson, "Voluntary Smiling Changes in Regional Brain Activity," *Psychological Science,* 4, 342-345.
7. Herbert Benson, M.D., *The Relaxation Response,* New York: William Morrow (1975)
8. H. G. Koenig, et al, "The relationship between religious activities and blood pressure in older adults," *International Journal of Psychiatry in Medicine* (1998) 28, 189-213.
9. E. McSherry, et al, "Spiritual Resources in older hospitalized men," *Social Compass,* (1987), 35 (4) p. 515-537.
10. T. E. Woods, et al, "Religiosity is associated with affective and immune status in symptomatic HIV infected men," *Journal of Psychosomatic Research*, 1998.

11. P. Pressman, et al, "Religious belief, depression and ambulatory status of women with broken hips," *American Journal of Psychiatry*, (1990), 147, 758-759.

12. R. Sudsuang, et al, "Effect of Buddhist meditation of serum cortisol and total protein levels, blood pressure, pulse rate, lung volume and reaction," *Physiology and Behavior*, (1991), 50, 543-548.

13. C. Alexander, et al, "Effects of Transcendental Meditation compared to other methods of relaxation and meditation in reducing risk factors such as hypertension, smoking, cholesterol," *Homeostasis*, 35, 243-264.

14. Herbert Benson, M.D., *The Relaxation Response.*

15. Herbert Benson, M.D., *The Relaxation Response.*

16. Jon Kabat Zinn, <u>*Full Catastrophe Living*</u>, New York, Bantam Doubleday Publishing Group, Inc. 1990.

17. Jon Kabat Zinn, <u>*Full Catastrophe Living*</u>

Chapter 4

1. Richard Davidson and Jon Kabat-Zinn, "Alterations in brain and immune function produced by mindfulness meditation," *Journal of Psychosomatic Medicine,* (2003) 65: 564-570.

2. Jon Kabat-Zinn, *Full Catastrophe Living.*

3. Jon Kabat-Zinn, Excerpts from *Meditation for Optimum Health,* Boulder, CO., Sounds True, 1999. Music licensed through Megatrax Production Music, Inc.

4. Lama Surya Das, *Awakening the Buddhist Heart*, New York, Broadway Books, (2000). 55, 60, 85-56, 154.

5. Jon Kabat-Zinn, Excerpts from *Meditation for Optimum Health*, Boulder, CO. Sounds True, 1999. Music licensed through Megatrax Production Music, Inc.

6. Woody Allen, *Quotations by Author*, July 27, 2008, http://www.quotationspage.com.

Chapter 5

1. Robert A Emmons and Joanna Hill, *Words of Gratitude,* Pennsylvania: Templeton Foundation Press, 2001, 7.

2. Emmons, 63.

3. M. E. McCullough, et al., "The grateful disposition: a conceptual and empirical topography," *Journal of Personality and Social Psychology*, 82, 112-127.

4. Emmons and Hill, quotes excerpted from *Words of Gratitude*, Music licensed by Megatrax Production Music, Inc.

Chapter 6

1. Thich Nhat Hanh, *The Miracle of Mindfulness*, Boston, Beacon Press, 1999, p. 15

2. Hanh, pp. 12, 65

3. John Lennon, *Quotations Page*, July 27, 2008, www.quotationspage.com/search.php3?homesearch=John+Lennon&startsearch=Search

4. Nadine Stair, *Quotations Page*, July 27, 2008, www.quotationspage.com/search.php3?Author=Nadine+Stair&file=other

5. Lama Surya Das, excerpt from *Awakening the Buddhist Heart*, New York: Random House, 2000. Music licensed by Megatrax Production Music, Inc.

6. Sogyal Rimpoche, *The Tibetan Book of Living and Dying*, New York: Harper Collins, 1993.

7. Jon Kabat-Zinn, *Full Catastrophe Living*, p. 288-290.

Chapter 7

1. Stephen Kosslyn, *Image and Brain*, Boston, MIT Press. 1996.

2. Hans Eysenck, "Personality, Stress and Disease," *Psychological Inquiry*, Vol. 2, Issue 3, 1991.

3. Anne Frank, Diary of a Young Girl, New York: Doubleday, 1967.

4. Carolyn Myss and Norman Shealy, M.D., *The Science of Medical Intuition*, 12-cassette audio series, Session 4, Boulder Colorado, Sounds True, 2002.

5. Myss, Session 4

6. Myss, Session 4

7. Myss, Session 4
8. Myss, Session 4
9. Brian Weiss, "Garden and staircase imagery," from *Meditation, Relaxation Regression,* CD, www.brianweiss.com. Music licensed by Megatrax Production Music, Inc.
10. Myss, Session 4
11. Myss, Session 4
12. Myss, Session 4

Chapter 8

1. Woody Allen, *Think-Exist,* July 7, 2008, www.thinkexist.com /quotes/Woody_Allen
2. 1 Corinthians 13:1
3. Sir JohnTempleton, *Agape Love: A Tradition Found in Eight World Religions*, Philadelphia and London; Templeton Foundation Press, (1999), 60
4. Templeton,17
5. Templeton,34; from the *Hadith*
6. Henry Wadsworth Longfellow, *Brainy Quote,* July 27, 2008, www.brainyquote.com/quotes/authors/h/heney_wadsworth_longfello.h tml.
7. James House [referenced in text].
8. Sir John Templeton, *Golden Nuggets,* Philadelphia and London, Templeton Foundation Press, (1997), 48
9. Victor Frankl, *Man's Search for Meaning*, New York, Simon & Schuster, 1959, 86
10. Sharon Salzberg, *Lovingkindness: The Revolutionary Art of Happiness,* Boston, Shambhala, (1998), 23.
11. D. Spiegel et al, "Effect of Psychosocial Treatment on Survival of Patients with Metastatic Breast Cancer," *Lancet* ii, (1989), pp. 888-91.
12. J. K. Kucolt-Glaser, et al "Psychosocial modification of immunocompetence in medical students," *Psychosomatic Medicine* 46, 7-14.

13. D. C. McClelland, "The Effect of Motivational Arousal through films on salivary Immunoglobulin A," *Psychology and Health* (1998) 2 31-52.
14. John O'Brunn, *Roseto Story: An Anatomy of Health*, (1979), University of Oklahoma Press
15. Deborah Kesten, Larry Scherwitz, The Enlightened Diet: 7 weight loss solutions that nourish body, mind and soul. Celestial Arts, 2007.

Chapter 9

1. Jack Kornfield, *Your Buddha Nature: Teachings on the Ten Perfections* (audio program). Boulder, Colorado, Sounds True, 1999. Kornfield, Jack.
2. Dalai Lama and Howard Cutler, *The Art of Happiness* (New York, Penguin Putnam, 1998) 179

Chapter 10

1. Woody Allen, *Quotations Page*, July 27, 2008, http://www.quotationspage.com/quotes/Woody_Allen
2 Helen Keller, *Quotations Page*, July 27, 2008, http://www.quotationspage.com/quotes/Hellen_Keller
3. Helen Keller, *Quotations Page*, July 27, 2008, http://www.quotationspage.com/quotes/Hellen_Keller
4. Lama Surya Das, *Awakening the Buddhist Heart*, (New York, Broadway Books, 2000), 182
5. Graham Green, *The Third Man* (New York, Penguin Putnam, 1999)
6. Helen Keller, *Quotations Page*, July 27, 2008, http://www.quotationspage.com/quotes/Hellen_Keller

Chapter 11

1. Christiane Northrup, *Your Diet, Your Health*, Audio Program, (Chicago, Heitz Wilson, Inc., MCMXCIX)
2. Northrop, Audio program

3. Ram Dass, *Still Here* (New York, Berkeley Publishing Group 2000) 85
4. Northrup, Audio program.
5. Donald F. Klein and Michael R. Liebowits, "Hysteroid Dysphoria," *Psychiatric Clinics of North America*, December 1979, 11:3
6. Northrup, Audio program.
7. Bob Schwartz, *Diets Don't Work*, (Houston, Breakthru Publishing, 1996
8. Molly Katzen, Interview for *Body and Soul Magazine*.

Chapter 12

1. Larry Dossey, M.D., *Reinventing Medicine,* New York, Harper Collins Publishers, 1999, 9
2. Bhante Walpola Piyananda, *Saffron Days in L.A,* Boston. Shambhala Publications, 2001. Forward by Dalai Lama.
3. Jawaharlal Nehru, *Wit and Wisdom of Jawaharlal Nehru,* Delhi, New Book Society of India, 1960, 264.
4. Sir John Templeton, *Agape Love,* Philadelphia & London, Templeton Foundation Press, 1999, 37
5. Larry Dossey, M.D., *Reinventing Medicine,* New York, Harper Collins Publishers 1999
6. Francis Crick, *The Astonishing Hypothesis: The Scientific Search for the Soul,* New York, Touchstone, 1995.
7. Ram Dass, 5
8. I. Regardie, *The Philosopher's Stone,* St. Paul: Llewellyn Publications, 1970, 90, Randolph Severson, "The Alchemy of Dreamwork: Reflections on Freud and Alchemic Tradition", Dragonflies (Spring 1979): 109
9. Dossey, 7
10. Mona Lisa Schultz, *Awakening Intuition*, New York, Three Rivers Press, 1998, 108.
11. Ram Dass, Preface, 1
12. Robert Van de Castel, *Our Dreaming Mind,* New York, Ballantine, 1994.

13. W. Braud, et al. "Electrodermal Correlates of Remote Attention: Autonomic Reactions to Unseen Gaze," Proceedings of the 33rd annual convention of the Parapsychological Association (1990), 14-28. W. Braud, "Human Interconnectedness: Research Indicators", Revision 14. no.3 (1992): 140-48; Marilyn Scholiz and Stephen LaBerge, "Covert Observation increases skin conductance in subjects unaware of when they are being observed: a replication," *Journal of Parapsychology* 61 (1997) 197-201.

14. Carol Adrienne, *The Purpose of Your Life,* New York, Eagle rook, An Imprint of William Morrow and Company, Inc. 1998, 108.

15. Adrienne, p.108

16. Edgar Mitchell, *The Way of the Explorer,* New York: G.P Putnam's Sons, 1996, 51.

17. Bernard R. Grad, "Some biological effects of laying on of hands: A review of experiments with animals and plants,'" *Journal of the American Society for Psychical Research,* (1960) 59a.

18. Grad, 59a.

19. Grad, 59a.

20. Grad, 59a.

21. B. Grad, R. J. Cadoret, and G. I. Paul, "The influence of an unorthodox method of wound healing in mice," *International Journal of Parapsychology,* 3(1961):5-24.

22. Rene Peoc'h, "Mise en evidence d'un effect psycho-physique chez l'hommeet la poussin sur le tycoscope," Doctoral thesis, University of Nantes, France, 1986

23. Randolph C Byrd, "Positive Therapeutic Effects of Intercessory Prayer in a Coronary Care Unit Population," *Southern Medical Journal* (1988) 81, no.7 826-9.

24. Fred Sicher, et al, "A Randomized Double Blind Study of the Effect of Distant Healing in a Population with Advanced AIDS: Report of a Small-Scale Study," *Western Journal of Medicine* (1998): 169, 6 356-63.

25. Sean O'Laoire, "An Experimental Study of the Effects of Distant Healing, Intercessory Prayer on Self Esteem, Anxiety and Depression," *Alternative Therapies,* (1887) 6 39-53.

26. David J. Muchsam, et al, "Effects of Qigong on Cell-Free Myosin Physphorylation: Preliminary Experiments," *Subtle Energies* 5, (1994): no I. 93-108.

27. Garrett L.Yount, M.D., et al "Cell Biology Meets Qigong." *Explorer: Newsletter of the Society for Scientific Exploration* (1997)13: 2, 3.

28. Dossey, 25

29. Eva Cassidy, *Songbird* CD, Track 5.

30. Rodney F. Falk, "The Death of Death with Dignity," *American Journal of Medicine* 77 (1984). 5 775-6.

31. Kathleen Dowling Singh, *The Grace in Dying*, San Francisco; Harper Collins, 1998.

32. Raymond Moody, *Life After Life,* San Francisco, Harper Collins, 2001.

33. Carolyn Myss, *Energy Anatomy*, Audio program, Boulder Colorado, Sounds True.

34. August L. Reader, III, "The Internal Mystery Plays: The Role of the Visual System in contemplative Practice," *Alternative Therapies I,* (1995). 4 54-63.

35. Brian Weiss, *Many Lives, Many Masters*, 1988, Simon & Schuster, Inc.: 1988.

36. Barbara Cooney, *Miss Rumphius*, New York, Puffin Books, 1982.

Bibliography

Achterberg, Jeanne. *Imagery in Healing: Shamanism and Modern Medicine.* Boston: Shambhala Publications, Inc. 1985.

Adrienne, Carol. *The Purpose of Your Life: Finding Your Place in the World Using Synchronicity, Intuition and Uncommon Sense.* New York: Eagle Brook An Imprint of William Morrow and Company, Inc., 1998.

Benson, Herbert, M.D. *The Relaxation Response.* New York: Harper Collins, 1976.

— *Timeless Healing: The Power and Biology of Belief.* New York: Fireside, a division of Simon & Schuster, Inc., 1997.

Benson, Herbert M.D. and Eileen M. Stuart, R.N., M.S. *The Wellness Book: The Comprehensive Guide to Maintaining Health and Treating Stress-Related Illness.* New York: A Fireside Book, Published by Simon & Schuster, 1992.

Boorstein, Sylvia. *It's Easier Than You Think: The Buddhist Way to Happiness.* New York. Harper San Francisco a trademark of Harper Collins Publishers, 1995.

— *Pay Attention, for Goodness' Sake: practicing the perfections of the heart the Buddhist path of kindness.* New York: Ballantine Books, 2002.

— *That's Funny, You Don't Look Buddhist: On Being a Faithful Jew and a Passionate Buddhist.* New York, Harper San Francisco, HarperCollins Publishers, Inc., 1997.

Borysenko, Joan, Ph.D. *Minding the Body, Mending the Mind.* New York: Bantam Books, published with arrangement with Addison Wesley Publications, Inc., 1987.

Borysenko, Joan, Ph.D. and Miroslav Borysenko, Ph.D. *The Power of the Mind to Heal: Renewing Body, Mind, and Spirit.* Carlsbad, CA: Hay House, Inc., 1994.

Brenner, Paul, M.D., Ph.D. *Buddha in the Waiting Room: Simple Truths About Health, Illness, and Healing.* Hillsboro, Oregon: Beyond Words Publishing, Inc. 2002.

Brussat, F., and M.A .Brussat. *Spiritual Rx: Prescriptions for living a meaningful life.* New York: Hyperion, 2000.

Casarjian, Robin. *Forgiveness: A Bold Choice for a Peaceful Heart.* New York: Bantam Books, 1992.

Chodron, Pema. *Comfortable with Uncertainty: 108 Teachings.* Boston, Shambhala, 2002.

— *Start Where You Are: A Guide to Compassionate Living.* Boston: Shambhala, 2001.

— *When Things Fall Apart: Heart Advice for Difficult Times.* Boston: Shambhala, 1997.

Chopra, Deepak M.D. *Quantum Healing: Exploring the Frontiers of Mind/Body Medical Meditation.* New York: Bantam Books, 1989.

Cooney, Barbara. *Miss Rumphius.* New York, Puffin Books, 1982.

Dalai Lama. *Ethics for the New Millennium.* New York: Riverhead Books, Published by The Berkley Publishing Group, a division of Penguin Putnam, Inc., 1999.

Dalai Lama and Howard C.Cutler, M.D. *The Art of Happiness: A Handbook for Living.* New York: Riverhead Books, a member of Penguin Putnam, Inc. 1998.

Dossey, Larry, M.D. *Reinventing Medicine: Beyond Mind-Body to a New Era of Healing.* New York: Harper Collins, 1999.

— *Healing Beyond the Body: Medicine and the Infinite Reach of the Mind Boston.* Shambhala Publications, Inc. 2001.

Dowling Singh, Kathleen. *The Grace in Dying: A Message of Hope, Comfort, and Spiritual Transformation,* San Francisco, Harper Collins, 2000.

Emmons, Robert A. and Joanna Hill. *Words of Gratitude: For Mind, Body, and Soul.* Radnor, Pennsylvania: Templeton Foundation Press, 2001.

Frankl, Victor. *Man's Search for Meaning.* New York, Simon & Schuster, 1959.

Grof, Stanislav, M.D. *The Holotropic Mind: The Three Levels of Human Consciousness and How They Shape Our Lives.* New York, Harper Collins Publishers, 1993.

Hample, Stuart and Marshall, Eric Children's Letters to God: The New Collection New York: Workman Publishing, 1991.

BIBLIOGRAPHY

Harvard Medical School. *Clinical Training in Mind/Body Medicine.* Boston: Mind Body
Medical Institute, October 29-November 2, 2001.

Heller, David, Ph.D. *Dear God: Children's Letters to God.* New York: A Perigee Book Published by the Berkley Publishing Group, 1987.

Khalsa, Dharma Singh, M.D. and Cameron Stauth. *Meditation as Medicine: Activate the Power of Your Natural Healing Force.* New York: Pocket Books, a division of Simon & Schuster, Inc., 2001.

Kornfield, Jack. *A Path with Heart; A Guide Through the Perils and Promises of Spiritual Life.* New York: Bantam Books, 1993.

— *After the Ecstasy, the Laundry: How the Heart Grows Wise on the Spiritual Path.* New York: Bantam Books, 2000.

— *The Art of Forgiveness, Lovingkindness, and Peace.* New York: Bantam Books, 2002.

— *Your Buddha Nature: Teachings on the Ten Perfections* (audio program). Boulder, Colorado, Sounds True, 1999.

Kosslyn, Stephen. *Image and Brain.* Boston, MIT Press. 1996.

Lama Surya Das. *Awakening the Buddha Within: Tibetan Wisdom for the Western World.* New York: Doubleday Books, 1997.

— *Awakening the Buddhist Heart: Integrating Love, Meaning, and Connection into Every Part of Your Life.* New York: Broadway Books, 2000.

— *Awakening to the Sacred: Creating a Personal Spiritual Life.* New York: Broadway Books, 1999.

— *Letting Go of the Person You Used to Be: Lessons on Change, Loss, and Spiritual Transformation.* New York: Broadway Books, 2003.

Marshall, Eric and Stuart Hample. *Children's Letters to God.* New York: Pocket Books, a division of Simon & Schuster, Inc., 1966.

Moody, Raymond A., M.D. *Life After Life.* New York: Bantam Books, a division of Bantam Doubleday Dell Publishing Group, Inc., 1976.

Muller, Wayne. *Legacy of the Heart: The Spiritual Advantages of a Painful Childhood.* New York, A Fireside Book Published by Simon &Schuster 1992.

Myss, Caroline, Ph.D. and C. Norman Shealy, ,M.D. *The Creation of Health: The Emotional, Psychological, and Spiritual Responses That Promote Health and Healing.* New York: Three Rivers Press, Member of the Crown Publishing Group, a division of Random House, Inc., 1988.

— *The Science of Medical Intuition: Self-Diagnosis and Healing with Your Body's Energy Systems.* (12-cassette audio program) Boulder, Co: Soundstrue, 2002.

Nehru, Jawaharlal. *Wit and Wisdom of Jawaharlal Nehru.* Delhi, New Book Society of India, 1960.

Northrup, Christiane, M.D. *Your Diet, Your Health* (audio program). Chicago: Heitz/Wilson, Inc. MCMXCIX.

— *Women's Bodies, Women's Wisdom: Creating Physical and Emotional Health and Healing.* New York: Bantam Books, 1998.

Orloff, Judith, M.D. *Intuitive Healing: 5 Steps to Physical, Emotional, and Sexual Wellness.* New York: Times Books, a division of Random House, Inc., 2000.

— *Second Sight: A Psychiatrist Clairvoyant Tells her Extraordinary Story.* New York: Warner Books, Inc., 1996

Piyananda, Bhante Walpola. *Saffron Days in L.A.* Boston. Shambhala Publications, 2001. Forward written by Dalai Lama.

— *Saffron Days in L.A.: Tales of a Buddhist Monk in America.* Boston: Shambhala Publications, Inc., 2001.

Prophet, Elizabeth Clare. *Reincarnation: The Missing Link in Christianity.* Corwin Springs, MT: Summit University Press, 1997.

Ram Dass. *Still Here: Embracing Aging, Changing, and Dying.* New York: Riverhead Books, Published by the Berkley Publishing Group, a division of Penguin Putnam Inc., 2000.

Rossman, Martin L. M.D. *Guided Imagery for Self-Healing: An Essential Resource for Anyone Seeking Wellness.* Novato, California: H. J. Kramer Book published in a joint venture with New World Library, 2000.

BIBLIOGRAPHY

Roth, Geneen. *Appetites: On the Search for True Nourishment.* New York: Penguin Putnam, Inc., 1997.

— *Feeding the Hungry Heart: The Experience of Emotional Eating.* New York: Penguin Putnam, Inc., 1993.

Sarley, Ila and Garrett. *Walking Yoga: Incorporate Yoga Principles into Dynamic Walking Routines for Physical Health, Mental Peace and Spiritual Enrichment.* New York: Fireside a trademark of Simon & Schuster, Inc., 2002.

Salzberg, Sharon. *A Heart As Wide as the World: Stories on the Path of Lovingkindness.* Boston: Shambhala Publications, Inc. 1997.

— *Faith: Trusting Your Own Deepest Experience.* New York: Riverhead Books, a member of Penguin Putnam, Inc., 2002.

— *Lovingkindness: The Revolutionary Art of Happiness.* Boston: Shambhala, 1997.

Schulz, Mona Lisa, M.D., Ph.D. *Awakening Intuition: Using Your Mind-Body Network for Insight and Healing.* New York: Random House, Inc., 1998.

Schwartz, Bob. *Diets Don't Work.* Houston, Breakthru Publishing, 1996.

Siegel, Bernie S., M.D. *Love, Medicine & Miracles.* New York: Harper Collins Publishers, Inc., 1990.

— *Peace, Love and Healing.* New York: Harper Publishers, 1989.

— *Prescriptions for Living: Inspirational Lessons for a Joyful, Loving Life.* New York: Harper Collins Publishers, 1990.

Sogyal Rinpoche. *The Tibetan Book of Living and Dying.* New York: Harper Collins Publishers, 1994.

Steindl-Rast, D. *Gratefulness, the heart of prayer.* New York: Paulist, 1984.

Talbot, Michael. *The Holographic Universe.* New York: Harper Collins Publishers, 1991.

Templeton, Sir John. *Agape Love: A Tradition Found in Eight World Religions.* Philadelphia: Templeton Foundation Press, 1999.

— *Golden Nuggets.* Philadelphia and London, Templeton Foundation Press, 1997.

Thich Nhat Hanh. *The Heart of the Buddha's Teaching: Transforming Suffering Into Peace, Joy, and Liberation.* New York: Broadway Books, 1998.

— *Living Buddha, Living Christ.* New York: Riverhead Books, Published by The Berkley Publishing Group, a division of Penguin Putnam, Inc., 1995.

— *The Miracle of Being Awake.* Boston. Beacon Press, 1975, 1976.

— *Teachings on Love.* Berkeley, California: Parallax Press, 1998.

— *Touching Peace: Practicing the Art of Mindful.* Living Berkeley, California: Parallax Press, 1992.

Andrew. *Eating Well for Optimum Health: The Essential Guide to Bringing Health and Pleasure Back to Eating.* New York: Quill, an imprint of Harper Collins Publishers, 2000.

Weiss, Brian L., M.D. *Many Lives, Many Masters: The True Story of a Prominent Psychiatrist, His Young Patient, and the Past-Life Therapy That Changed Both Their Lives.* New York: A Fireside Book, Published by Simon & Schuster, Inc., 1988.

— *Messages from the Masters: Tapping into the Power of Love.* New York: Warner Books, Inc., 2000.